The Lighter Side of Breast Cancer Recovery

Lessons Learned Along the Path to Healing

Tammy A. Miller

First Edition

Hugz and Company
Lighthearted Press
530 Hillside Ave.
State College, PA 16803
www.hugzandcompany.com

Copyright© 2004 Tammy A. Miller
All rights reserved

This book, or parts thereof, may not be reproduced in any form without permission.

ISBN 0-9701379-3-1

Printed in the United States of America

*Dear Lord, please use me this day
beyond my wildest dreams!*

This book is dedicated to
all the special people who
have crossed my path
and touched my life.

The Lighter Side of Breast Cancer Recovery

Lessons Learned Along the Path to Healing

From professional clown to breast cancer survivor, this is the story of one woman's journey looking for the lighter side of breast cancer recovery.

"When your heart over-flows, so do your eyes. Whether it is happiness or sadness, they both work the same."

Contributed by Humor Team member
Christina Guyer
10/12/01

Acknowledgments

There are so many people who worked to make this book happen and I want thank them all!

To my beautiful daughters, Lacey and Tiffany. Girls, we have been through a lot together, but God has provided us with so many blessings, and always brings us through to the sunshine. I love you more than you could possibly know! To my family, my mother, Ruth, my partner Charlie (CJ), my father, Jim, my brothers, Jim and Mike, and many other family members who were there to support me along the way. There is really no way that words on a page could express how much gratitude I have for all of you for everything you have done for me. From love when I needed it most, to understanding and support on the great days, and less than great days, to your financial assistance to make this book happen. Each day I thank God for giving me your loving presence. You are the greatest - I thank you all and love you!

To my dear, "pinky swear" friend, Mary. Mary, we both know your Mom and God worked out quite a plan to bring us together in this crazy world of clowning! I thank God each day for you and the blessings you have brought to my life. You truly are an "Angel". I love it when a plan comes together!

My friends, I thank you for sharing all the "positives" along the journey. Each day I am thankful that my life is so full of wonderful people, including some of the best friends in the world! You were there when I needed you most with support, love, food, and even snow shoveling when I was unable to do it!!! To all of the friends that I have been blessed with, I thank you.

To the members of my Humor Team, you took the responsibility of laughter very seriously! Thank you for looking for the brightest side of everything as we walked along the path together! Thank you for helping me to personally understand the healing power of laughter. I wish each and every one of you many blessings as you walk your own path in life.

To Aaron Bleznak for saving my life. You went above and beyond "your job" to show compassion and concern for me as your patient. In the words of one of your favorite philosophers, Peter Parker, "With power comes great responsibility". I thank you for taking on the responsibility to help breast cancer patients, and for being there when I needed you the most along my path to healing.

To all of the wonderful healthcare providers that God placed on my path. I know that this is "your job", but the love and compassion that you showed went beyond the job and was so greatly appreciated. Thank you for making this journey more bearable!

To all the people at ARL and Advanced Color Graphics who helped me with the computer-related questions. This project would have been a great deal more difficult without your expertise. Thank you for making me "look good".

To all the people who prayed for me as I traveled on this journey. Thank you for keeping me lifted in prayer through the big concerns as well as the "teeny-tiny" concerns! Our God truly is an AWESOME God – thank you for your love!

Table of Contents

Lessons learned 1-2
Cast of characters 3
Introduction 4-7

Chapters

1	Beginning the Journey	8-13
2	Meeting with Dr. B	14-17
3	Surgery Number One	18-25
4	The Diagnosis and Prognosis	26-31
5	Hiring the "H Team"!	32-39
6	The Waiting Days	40-61
7	A Truly WILD party!!	62-67
8	Pennies from Heaven	68-71
9	How to Tell Others	72-77
10	The "Big" Surgery	78-91
11	Just call me Dolly	92-97
12	Office Visits	98-101
13	Signs from God	102-109
14	A Very Difficult Decision	110-119
15	Becoming a Hyster Sister	120-127
16	Another Very Special Party	128-131
17	A Few "Normal" Responses	132-137
18	When I am Radiated, I Shall Wear Purple	138-153
19	The RAG Party!!	154-157
20	Winning the Mind Game	158-164

Appendix

Suggested questions 165-171
References 120-127
Red Nose Fund 175
Need a Speaker? 176-178
Other books by Lighthearted Press 179
Photo Section 180-182

Before I start with my actual story of recovery, I would like to offer this list of 20 very important lessons that I learned along the path to recovery. I will look at each of these lessons in greater detail as we progress through the book.

These are lessons I believe anyone can use, whether they are facing breast cancer, other cancers, illnesses, or any other of the challenges that life throws our way. These lessons serve as a reminder that we have choices in how we deal with whatever comes our way.

I prefer to call these lessons, as this journey was a journey of learning. I learned about myself. I learned about others. And, I learned, most importantly, that I could play a major role in the tone of my recovery.

I ask that you walk with me down my path to recovery, and embrace these lessons and make them your own.

20 Lessons Learned Along the Path

Lesson One – Don't put off your yearly exams. Make the call – schedule the appointment.

Lesson Two – Trust your own instincts.

Lesson Three – Keep a record of everything that is happening.

Lesson Four – Develop a personal mantra to replace negative thoughts.

Lesson Five – Recruit your personal Humor Team! (No cost involved!)

Lesson Six – Be prepared to put up your own personal shield of protection.

Lesson Seven– Start and keep a "Recovery File".

Lesson Eight – Find love and laughter everywhere.

Lesson Nine –Tell your closest family and friends of your diagnosis in person.

Lesson Ten – Be informed!

Lesson Eleven– Remain positive in every single way that you can – no matter how small.

Lesson Twelve - Write down the questions that you want to ask.

Lesson Thirteen– Look for the smallest blessings in each day.

Lesson Fourteen – Know that you have choices.

Lesson Fifteen – Remember, you are a unique person!

Lesson Sixteen – Celebrate the smallest victories.

Lesson Seventeen– Accept that there are some things in life we cannot change.

Lesson Eighteen– Keep your doctors and health care providers accountable.

Lesson Nineteen – Thank your healthcare providers.

Lesson Twenty – Live life to the fullest!

A Quick Reference for the "Cast of Characters"

Since I refer to the doctors in this story by the first letter of their last name, I will provide you with a "key" to the names for quick reference:

Dr. G – Initially read the mammogram at the Breast Care Center and detected a possible problem; advised against a needle biopsy for certainly; performed the pre-surgery procedures

Dr. B – My surgeon for the first two surgeries and my follow-up cancer doctor

Dr. M – The Anesthesiologist who performed the pre-surgery procedure

Dr. V – The Anesthesiologist in the operating room

Dr. W – The Oncology doctor

Dr. C – The OB-GYN doctor who performed the hysterectomy

Dr. D – The Radiation/Oncology doctor

Introduction

"Sometimes the only sense we can make out of life is a sense of humor." — Unknown author

The goal of this publication is two-fold. The first purpose is to help other people who may have recently been diagnosed with breast cancer, are recovering from breast cancer, or have a family member or friend facing the challenges that a breast cancer diagnosis can bring to their lives. The second purpose is to serve as a personal reminder of my experiences, and the wonders and beauty of life.

Breast cancer is certainly no laughing matter. In fact, I have chosen the lighter side not in any way, shape or form because I do not take breast cancer seriously, but quite the contrary. I have chosen to look at the lighter side because it IS so serious. This whole journey has forced me to reflect upon my life – past, present and future, and it puts a whole new spin on the idea that sometimes the only sense we can make out of life is a sense of humor.

When I was diagnosed with breast cancer at age 42, I was a professional clown, a motivational speaker and workshop presenter, and I had recently started my own company. I also worked as a trainer at a large university with over 18 years of training experience. In many of my presentations, I helped people understand the value of a positive attitude and how we can use humor to deflect some of the most difficult situations. When I was diagnosed, I knew that it was time to put my own words into action and look at how I was personally going to deal with the situation that I had just been handed. I may have been a trained clown, but I know that you don't need to be a clown – or even have a great sense of humor – to take positive steps, sometimes very small steps, that make a significant difference in how you respond to life and those around you. In this particular case, I further discovered that your recovery and quality of life can, in a large part, be determined by how you CHOOSE to embrace the situation.

Since I do a lot of presentations, I always say that everything in my life is simply speech material. I pull from personal experiences to make my presentations stronger. Prior to my diagnosis I certainly felt that I had ample material from which to draw. However, God had another plan. In later chapters, I discuss how I have come to a better understanding of this "wrinkle on the road", and again realize that, for everything in life, there is a reason.

In dealing with my own breast cancer, I learned that there CAN be a *Lighter Side to Breast Cancer Recovery*, and it can be an important coping tool that lifts your spirits, builds your body, and keeps you going in even the toughest of times.

This book is not intended to be a technical reference manual to breast cancer, there are a lot of good books out there already for this purpose, many of them I reference in the Reference Section. This book is designed to be a story of one woman's journey (mine), and a look at one method to cope and recover from what can be a devastating diagnosis. Although there are a few technical parts, the story as a whole is intended to be more of a celebration of life, and to offer of an option to recovery.

I wrote this book to share the many lessons that I learned with other women who may be recovering from breast cancer, but many of the lessons can also be applied to surviving other challenges in life. It is also my hope that not only can the individual affected be lifted by this information, but also her or his family members and friends as well.

There are some parts of this book that are a little graphic in nature and may be offensive to some. This is certainly not the intention, but in telling this story, I felt it necessary to offer a more thorough description of events as they transpired. I would like to thank all of the special people who read this material as it was growing into a real book. I hope with more than one set of eyes, we were able to correct the most blatant of grammar and spelling errors. In the event we missed any, I do apologize to you as the reader.

Throughout this book, I also have included sections relating to "questions to ask" and positive thoughts and words. You may or may not find this information helpful, but I have tried to look for the brighter side in everything that was happening in my life. Sometimes it was very easy to see this side, especially when I looked through my own "Recovery Folder", and other times I had to try a little harder to see the lighter and brighter side.

In a later chapter, I spend a lot of time describing my Humor Team and the valuable role they played in my recovery. One of my team members reminded me early on that "I was no longer in control of my life, but life was controlling me. I was being told where to go, when to go and what was going to happen when I got there." I reflected on her words for a while and was reminded of the saying I use so many times with my family, friends and in workshops I present, "You cannot change other people, you can only change how you respond to other people". I realized that this was the same situation but with different terms. <u>I knew first of all and most importantly that I have choices</u>!!! If I chose to follow the most effective path to recovery I would have to lose some of my stubborn independence and rely on others. I could not change what was happening; I could only change how I responded to the situation.

Throughout it all, the greatest lesson I have learned is that there is great healing power in love and laughter. From my own personal faith in God, to the many small celebrations of life, to the valuable lessons that my own Humor Team taught me during a difficult time - I am forever grateful and very thankful!!!

It is my most heartfelt desire that by sharing this story and embracing the ideas in this book, your life, or the life of those you love will somehow be more positive. Whether it is breast cancer recovery, or any other challenge you face in your life, I pray you will indeed be better equipped and able to find the Lighter Side of Recovery. Wishing you many blessing!

Now, on with the story...

Lesson One - *Don't put off your yearly exams. Use your birthday as a good reminder, and if you can't remember your own birthday, check that birth certificate and write it down. There are times when we have to be a little forceful in asking for an appointment, but be persistent and MAKE THE CALL – SCHEDULE THE APPOINTMENTS!!!*

During the month of October for Breast Cancer Awareness Month, many areas offer special programs, including free mammograms. If this is a concern of yours, please check with your healthcare providers for additional information.

Breast cancer is not strictly a "women's disease". According to the 2003 statistics from the American Cancer Society, about 1200 new cases of breast cancer are diagnosed in American men each year (compared to about 200,000 cases of breast cancer in U.S. women).

Chapter One
Beginning the Journey

"The world is full of suffering. It is also full of the overcoming of it." — Helen Keller

My personal journey started on September 14, 2001. Personally, I won't call it a battle, more of a journey, or going down a path of unknown destination, but you must use your own phraseology for comfort.

Actually, it had started a few months before when I noticed my once perky nipple decided it wanted to turn into an "inny". I noticed a collapse that seemed to be getting deeper as the weeks went on. I was adamant about getting the recommended female exam every year around my birthday (this seemed to be the least painful and less taxing on the brain to remember each year). I figured as long as I could remember when my birthday was, I could remember to get the exam.

On July 12 (my birthday is actually July 22, for any of you card-crazy people out there!) I went to the doctor's office for the check-up. I usually saw the Physician's Assistant, since she was the only female in the office, so this visit was no different.

I told her right away about the perky traitor that decided to turn "inny" on me. She felt the breast and said that she didn't see anything to be concerned about (boy, was she wrong!). Since she didn't see any reason for concern, she wasn't in a hurry to make a mammogram appointment, and said I could do it whenever I got a chance. The pap went fine and I told her I would call for the mammogram appointment later in the week. She indicated that there was no hurry and I told her I would rather stay regular with my appointment, so I would make the arrangements. It took a little over two months to get an appointment for a mammogram. See Lesson One – be persistent!

On Friday, September 14, 2001, I arrived at the local Breast Care Center for the mammogram. Women have individual experiences with a mammogram. For some, there is pain due to the squishing of the breast. Maybe squish is a harsh word, but it seems to me to be the most accurate! For others, there is slight discomfort. Let's face it, they are taking a body part and making it one third of its natural size so, yes, there is discomfort associated with this process. Yet, others don't feel much of anything. I haven't personally met any of those women, but the statistics show they do exist. Whatever your level of pain or discomfort, it lasts less than five minutes, and can truly save your life – it is worth the time and effort!! Back to Lesson One!

I am one of the women who feel some slight discomfort. The process went quickly and I went on my merry way. I look back now and realize how very close I was to canceling that mammogram appointment. I was leaving town to visit my mother in Ohio and attend a family reunion, and I wanted to leave a day early, but decided I should stay the extra day and not cancel the mammogram. I am so thankful now that I kept THAT appointment!

I went on my visit to Ohio and returned Sunday night. On Monday I received a call that there was "an area of distortion" on my mammogram and they wanted me to come in for another check. I thought it simply meant that one of the films was messed up and they just wanted another Kodak moment with my breasts.

Since this was a follow-up to an abnormal mammy (by this time we all know what it is called so let's shorten it to mammy) the follow-up exam was scheduled for Thursday of that week, September 20, 2001.

Meeting Dr. G

When I arrived, I went through the usual "undress from the waist up, put the gown on and wait in the booth until we call your name". The technician came to get me and the appropriate photos were taken. I was just hoping they got my good side. The technician then took me into another room to meet with a doctor to get an ultrasound. Hmm, this wasn't going the same way they usually do – I knew something was not quite right.

I jumped up onto the table as instructed. All right I know you can't "jump" in those gowns without falling out, so I gingerly stepped on the step stool and "scooched" onto the table! The doctor arrived; I will refer to him as Dr. G to maintain his privacy. He was a good-looking guy so I thought, "Well, the time spent isn't a complete loss," and he indicated that the mammy had actually picked up something that he wanted to check out with the ultrasound. I still wasn't concerned.

He did the ultrasound on the "inny" breast and asked me to go ahead and put the gown back on so we could talk about the results. I didn't even realize I was only half dressed. What he was doing was really interesting. In fact, the whole process was really interesting; I just wish we were talking about someone else!!

He showed me the film from the previous year and what they were picking up on the current mammy. There was a small area circled that was the area of concern. Had it not been circled, I don't know that I would have even noticed the difference. It didn't look like a lump or bump, but more like a tiny explosion on the film. He told me he didn't know exactly what he was looking at, but knew that if he took a needle biopsy and it came back negative he really wouldn't believe the results. Thank goodness he was a doubter!!! He told me he wanted me to see a surgeon and he expected the surgeon to suggest a surgical biopsy to see exactly what we were dealing with in the "inny" breast.

I mentioned that I had gone to see a Dr. B for another unrelated question a few years ago, and though I had only seen him briefly some time ago, I thought I would go back to see him. Dr. G told me that he had a great deal of respect for Dr. B and he was one of the best. That certainly gave me a little more comfort coming from one breast guy about another.

When I mentioned that I had noticed the change from perky to "inny" over the past year, he expressed his concern that we might be looking at a small cancer under the nipple that was pulling it in. Okay, okay, he now had my full attention and I had passed the threshold from a casual observer to an actively involved concerned participant.

He said the results would go to Dr. B's office and I could make an appointment to see him as soon as possible. There was a little bit of trouble going through the telephone tangle maze, but hey, we all deal with the "Press One or Two or Three or Forty-five syndrome!" After finally getting that taken care of I had the necessary appointment with Dr. B for five days later.

The "Pinky Swear"

When I went back to work after the ultrasound and realized that things may be changing in my life, I stopped to see one of my best friends and made her take a "pinky swear". If any of you out there don't know what that is, let me explain. You curl your little pinky with another person's pinky and make a "swear" about something. Does this sound juvenile to you? Yes, it is something from grade school, but for me at this time I needed her support. The pinky swear that we made was that if this turned out to be something bad, she had to swear to me that there would be no pity and she would do her very best to keep me laughing throughout the coming months.

This tiny gesture served as a wonderful reminder to both of us over the next few days that if it was a "biggie" diagnosis, we both understood that we couldn't change it and I really, really needed her there for support, positive encouragement, and laughter.

The time between Thursday and Tuesday was spent thinking, reflecting, and talking, but most importantly, WRITING down the questions I wanted to ask during my upcoming appointment with Dr. B. <u>Writing down</u> the questions is one area where I cannot emphasize the importance enough. I personally found a lot of information available through the internet. With this situation, and many others, there is a ton of information out there and you have to sift through to find out what has merit and what does not.

If you are dealing with a similar situation and do not have computer access, you can always check out the library or ask someone to assist you with this research. No matter what level of knowledge you are coming in at, you owe it to yourself to understand what is happening in your body. This knowledge will help you to not only understand what is happening in your body, but also what the doctors are telling you, and most importantly, as we will discuss in much greater detail later, being informed allows you to make your own decisions.

As you may know, October is Breast Cancer Awareness month across the nation. It seemed that everywhere I went there were pink ribbons and posters about breast cancer awareness. Trust me; at this point I was VERY aware of breast cancer, yet so thankful for that awareness as I believe it did indeed save my life!! If I had not pushed to have the tests done, the outcome could have been completely different, and you may not have had the opportunity to read this fascinating (tee-hee) book!

Lesson Two - *Trust your own instincts. If you think something is wrong, check it out with more than one source, and continue checking until you are sure of the results. When in doubt, check it out, again and again if necessary, with multiple sources.*

Chapter One
Meeting With Dr. B

"The bridge to success is never crossed alone."
— Unknown Author

When I arrived at Dr. B's place I was taken to the examination room and tried to ready myself for his exam. The room was very, very cold. I live in Pennsylvania and there was a seasonal Pennsylvania weather change going on outside, and the battle of the heat vs. air conditioner was in full swing.

When Dr. B (another really good looking guy, so maybe this wasn't going to be TOO bad!) arrived, I told him that if he wanted to see the difference in my breasts, and the "inny", he sure chose the wrong room. Even the "inny" was now standing at full attention from the cold! This seemed to break any possible ice (almost literally) that was in the room and the exam got started in the right direction. As it turned out, I didn't have to worry about that as Dr. B made me feel very comfortable from the beginning.

Dr. B did the usual exam and started with his questions. He asked what I had already been told by the doctor at the Breast Care Center. After I told him about the experience with Dr. G, he seemed pleased and said that all of the information I was told was correct. I liked the fact that he asked me what I had already been told so we didn't have to cover that ground twice.

I then started with my own list of questions. (There is a sample suggested list for your use in a later chapter, in case you really aren't sure what to ask.) He patiently listened and responded to each and every one of the questions, no matter how complex or simple. I never once felt rushed by this man, and that is so important to building confidence in your doctor.

He told me he wanted to do a surgical biopsy as soon as possible and he would most likely know on that day what we were dealing with. He explained exactly what he would be doing with the procedure in detail, even going so far as to draw a picture on a flipchart hanging in the exam room. I was as prepared as possible and we ended the first of our many meetings.

From this initial consultation, he also gave me a very important piece of advice. He said that I most likely would not remember everything he was going to say, so along with someone to take me home, make sure I brought a tape recorder and/or a camcorder to record the conversation. I chose the camcorder and I am so glad that I did. If you don't own one, borrow or rent one. A lot of people have them and they are rather inexpensive to rent. He was right. Although I was awake after the biopsy, it turned out to be a great reference when I was trying to remember exactly what he had said.

We concluded by setting up an outpatient appointment for the biopsy about two weeks later. This was all happening too quickly for my mind to comprehend! I do workshops and training, and I had been scheduled to present on the subject of managing interruptions in your life. WOW! I had just been handed what could and ultimately did result in a major interruption in my life! I called to have another instructor take my place on the day of my biopsy and I went home to think, and tried not to worry about the upcoming procedure.

Each person deals with this type of news in her own way. For me, I knew I could not change what was going on inside of Inny (yes, I might as well capitalize it, as I came to call it by this name of affection). So, I asked Dr. B to give me the information I needed and help me make the right decisions. On this he promised, and that helped build that important trust I was gaining in his attitude. I was praying that his skills matched his attitude, patience, and bedside manner.

Lesson Three – Keep a record of what is happening. One of the most important pieces of advice I was given came from my doctor (Dr. B). He told me to bring a tape recorder or a camcorder, if available, especially when I had surgery. When you come out from under the sedation, your mind isn't always clear. I chose a camcorder, and it worked great! There are so many questions, new terms used, and decisions to make. It was helpful to be able to go back and listen to what the doctor had said. If you do not own one, ask around, maybe a friend or family member has one to loan you. If not, they can be rented for a small cost. Whatever you have to do, they are well worth the investment.

Chapter Three
Surgery Number One

"God understands our prayers even when we can't find the words to say them."
— *Unknown Author*

    The day of the biopsy I arrived with my partner, I will refer to him as CJ from this point on, and camera in hand. No, CJ wasn't in my hand, but the camera was – well, you get the idea! I was told that Dr. B had an emergency at the hospital and would be at least an hour late. I wasn't too concerned since I had the whole day off and decided that if "I" were the emergency, I would certainly want Dr. B to take the time to care for me. When you try to put yourself in someone else's shoes it sometimes makes the waiting a bit easier.

    I was taken to the room and asked the usual questions about not eating or drinking for so many hours before I came in. Everyone in the outpatient area was very nice and the initial "stuff" went fine. From there I went back to see Dr. G in the Breast Care Center. Due to the type of lump (as I learned later, almost all of the growths are called lumps, whether a mass or actual lump) the idea was for Dr. G and his assistant to give me another mammy to pinpoint the exact location of the suspicious area. This time it was a little different.

    The technician brought me into another room at the Center where we met Dr. G. I was placed in a very straight back chair and wheeled into the mammogram machine. There I was positioned into the machine and squished again. The most difficult part this time was that I had to remain perfectly still AND SQUISHED for almost three minutes while they checked the film to make sure it was okay. Believe me, while being squished, three minutes sure seems like a lot longer than 180 seconds!

Then the fun stuff! (Before I tell you the specifics of the next medical procedure, I want to emphasize that it was the lighthearted interchange I had with the doctor and nurse during the procedure which made the experience tolerable.) Dr. G numbed Inny – I felt a little pressure but no pain as he used a needle to get her nice and numb. He then stuck a little funnel with a sharp hollow needle at the end into the top of Inny!!! From there he took another long needle (more like a piece of flexible wire) and stuck it into the funnel and into the breast. In reality it was probably 3-4 inches long, but seemed like a lot longer on the picture they sent to Dr. B. There was a series of four pictures taken. This was very important for Dr. B to be able to see exactly where he should make the cut and look for the suspicious tissue.

Dr. G and the technician were joking with me the entire time about the procedure. For some of you this may seem a bit cold, but I can honestly tell you that their lighthearted approach made all of the difference in my approach to the matter. Although this was a very serious situation, I kept remembering that I could not change it and I recalled the tremendous value the role of laughter can make in improving health.

Through all of the initial mammys and this procedure, the doctor made comments about my breasts being so dense. Personally, I didn't think he knew me well enough to make that personal judgment, but maybe he's just quick!!! The fact that I am petite (no, I never use the word *small* when it comes to my height or breast size!!!) but have dense breasts made it even more difficult for Dr. G to insert the needle. However, he did an excellent job of numbing me first and except for a little pressure I didn't feel much of anything. The procedure took maybe 20 minutes all together. They placed a hard surgical mask, similar to what you use when working with paint, over my breast and I was taken back to the room to wait for Dr. B.

As it turned out, he was close to two hours late for my surgery due to an emergency. I was ready to get this over with, but again, I felt that if I was the person who really needed his surgical skills, I would be happy he was there for me.

When Dr. B finally arrived in my room, he was wearing the traditional green scrubs, but it was his head covering that drew my attention!! When was the last time you met a guy wearing a bright blue cap with neon, hot pink triangles??? I knew I liked him from the beginning, but since I love bright colors – he was my kind of doctor!

He again patiently explained the procedure and asked if I had any questions. Since he did a thorough job preparing me for what was coming, I didn't have any questions. (Trust me, I made up for it later!! I think I broke his record for questions!) He told me he would see me after the surgery and we would talk more then. The nurse came back into the room and jacked up the I.V. and we were ready to roll. Shortly thereafter I was wheeled into the operating room.

I remember being moved from one table to the next, but that is all I remember until I woke up at the end of the surgery. When the anesthesiologist had talked to me before the surgery, he had explained that he was doing a local I.V. for the operation. I wouldn't feel anything and wouldn't be completely asleep, but if I did feel any pain, I was to let him know. I vaguely remember feeling a pinch a couple of times and I think he turned up the juice and I fell asleep on my own.

I woke up just as they were finishing the surgery. I remember hearing Dr. B talking to other people and then I was wheeled into the room to wake up completely.

About ten minutes later Dr. B came into the room. We had the video camera ready and again, I am very thankful for this important suggestion. He told me that he was very suspicious of the tissue he took out, and would be very surprised, happy, but surprised if the tissue came back cancer-free. He explained the hardness of the tissue and how this was a good indictor of non-healthy tissue, but he wouldn't know anything for certain for two days. I had an appointment to see him two days later to learn the actual results.

I was sent home to recover and think about the options ahead. It truly helped that he told me what he thought. Even though I had that glimmer of hope that he could be wrong, at least thinking that it probably was cancer helped me to make some decisions about what I might have to do in the very near future.

For some people, the idea of him telling me that there was a real possibility of cancer, without knowing for sure, was a bad decision on his or my part. Unless he was 100% sure, why should he tell me this and have me worry about the true news for a couple of days. However, I had developed a deep trust in Dr. B as a skilled surgeon. I knew that he was experienced in these matters, and I believed he would not tell me in this manner unless he was confident in his suspicion. I cannot emphasize enough how important it is to have faith in your caregivers!

First Tears

The ride home was the first time I cried, but I really didn't cry, more like my eyes leaked. I believe my only words on the way home were, "Now, how the hell (excuse the language) am I going to tell the girls (my daughters) THIS?" I don't live far from the hospital, but it was a long, quiet fifteen-minute ride. I quietly said a few other choice words, but not in anger, more in shock at this point.

The recovery at home went well. I used ice packs and some medication for pain that evening and went to work for most of the next day. I had to teach a class that night and a workshop early the following morning. For me, this was a good way to keep busy and try to make the time to the Thursday appointment go much faster.

I spent a lot of time reading and re-reading the books that the doctor had given me and the information I had found when searching the internet. This helped with the second, much longer list of questions I wanted to ask during the next appointment. One internet site I found extremely helpful was the National Institutes of Health, National Cancer Institute (www.nih.gov). I have used this site many times since then, not only to answer my questions, or find information that prompted more questions, but also to help others seeking information on cancers and other illnesses.

A lot of time was spent talking to family and friends about their thoughts. I didn't want to talk to other people who had been through this, as I didn't want someone saying something that would take away from the high level of trust I had personally developed in my doctor. The time was spent more in telling people that I needed their strength to support me when I was down, and how very important their role was on my Humor Team (more about that coming up). I wanted them to realize that they were a hand-chosen group of people. The team would not have any negative people as that is proven to slow recovery. Their ability to share love and laughter was going to be vital in my recovery.

Building My Shield

I mentioned in the "Lessons I Learned Along the Path" section about talking with others about what you are going through. It truly seemed like everyone had a sister, or a cousin, or a friend, who had gone through this and asked me if I wanted to talk with them about their ordeal. From the very beginning I learned to simply say "NO, thank you". Some people felt that I thought my experience was much worse than the one they knew about, and that was the reason why I didn't want to talk to their person. Others thought I was being rude, or something else. I reflected on why I was so adamant about NOT talking to others about the journey at this point. I am not normally a rude or nasty person, so I felt there had to be something else going on in my mind that I was closing people out. However, I wasn't shutting them out from supporting me; I just didn't want to hear any negative stories that would affect my positive attitude.

There are a lot of great support groups out to help people cope with a breast cancer diagnosis, treatments, and related feelings. For example the *Reach for Recovery, I Can Cope, and Look Good, Feel Better* programs, all offered through the American Cancer Society, are all excellent, if you feel you need support for you and your family. Only YOU can make this determination as to what you need.

After a great deal of reflection, I realized that what I was doing was actually PROTECTING MYSELF. In fact, I came to refer to it as "my shield of protection", or simply "my shield". My shield was protecting me from anyone or anything that was going to put the slightest negative thought in my head. It had been a few days since I had an overwhelming feeling that I was dealing with cancer, and I was actually "okay" with what was happening. I certainly did not like it, but I was dealing with the situation.

I cannot emphasize enough that at this point I could not change what was going on inside of my body, but I certainly could change how I looked at the journey and how I was going to respond. Negative thoughts can be placed so easily in our subconscious, and mostly by innocent comments being made like, "Well, I don't know if what you are being told is the best advice...", or one of my favorites, "Now, I know this won't happen to you, but let me tell you about the awful experience my (fill in the blank) had when she was dealing with breast cancer", or something to that effect. I said before that I had the utmost confidence in Dr. B and I was going to protect myself at all cost. Let's face it, he was the head of my humor and recovery team, and I was going into surgery knowing that this man was going to be a key part to my survival! I know that God was going to be guiding him during the surgery, but he was my human link to the beginning of the true cancer-free recovery. Don't be afraid to be polite and build your own shield!

Lesson Four –Develop a personal mantra and use it to replace any negative thought that squeezes its way into your head. This can be a single word, a phrase, a short song, whatever works for YOU to replace the negative with the positive. Remember, your brain can only process one thought at a time. Don't waste your brainpower on the negatives!

Chapter Four
The Diagnosis and Prognosis

"A mind once stretched by a new idea never regains its original dimensions."
- Oliver Wendall Holmes

On Thursday, October 11, 2001, I was scheduled to meet with Dr. B to discuss the test results. I had asked CJ, and my "pinky swear" friend, Mary to accompany me for a variety of reasons. First, for moral support, second, I felt that maybe a male and female perspective would offer a different interpretation of what the doctor was saying, and third to ask any questions they could think of that I might have missed. Keep in mind, this can be a very trying time and although we think of a thousand things to say before we get there, sometimes our minds just go blank.

My appointment was not until 1:00 in the afternoon, and I can tell you that the morning seemed to last forever. I had purposely scheduled a long meeting at work so that I knew my mind would be occupied elsewhere for at least a little time while I waited for the "moment of truth".

At the appointed time we arrived in the doctor's office, camera in hand, and clown noses in my bag. I already realized that this meeting would not be all cheery and sweet, so I brought the noses along as a supportive measure. I wasn't sure who needed it more, my team, the doctor, or me! I didn't know him very well, but I knew I wasn't going to be the usual patient – I had already hired members of my Humor Team, but more about that later!!!

I didn't think I was really nervous until I had to wait for Dr. B to arrive in the room. It took almost 25 minutes, but that 25 minutes may as well have been 250! I was in the examining room by myself, until my companions were summoned and I think I looked at every square inch of the room. I lay down, I sat up, I counted the number of tongue depressors in the canister (16 if you would like to know). I was really working up the nerve bunnies when Dr. B arrived. I told him I had people with me and the camera, so please don't say anything yet. I was so afraid of missing something really important in the exchange.

He laughed and said, "Okay, okay, just let me take a look at you for a minute." Ahh, that was so sweet, well, it was until I realized he meant the bandage covering my left breast!! Of course I knew that was what he meant, remember, it was stressful waiting!! (Looking back, the whole scene was almost surreal and like something from a comedy film. Hmmm, a film of my life – I wonder who they would get to play me? Maybe I can check with Dolly Parton, as she is one of my favorites! There might have to be a few, or at least a couple (wink-wink) costume adjustments needed, but she would be able to play the role very well!!)

He said everything looked good and he asked the nurse to go summon my companions and that he would be right back. Closer to the moment of truth – hurry up, let's get on with it!! When everyone was seated, camera rolling, he began. For the next 36 minutes (one of the advantages of having it taped – it has a timer), he calmly and thoroughly told me the diagnosis and answered every question I had. If your doctor does not do this, tell him or her that you really need to have the opportunity to talk and ask questions, and most importantly, have them answered to YOUR satisfaction. Make sure your doctor explains everything, AND in language you can understand. If you don't know the definition of the terms he or she uses – don't stop asking questions until you do. No matter how minor you think the questions are, remember, this is YOUR body and YOUR life.

I knew Dr. B was very busy, and I didn't want to waste his time, but we were talking about my LIFE. I wasn't just a patient, but a real live person who had a cancer growing in her breast. I needed to know what was going on and I needed to know now. There was never one second that I felt Dr. B was rushing me, or his responses (another part of my thankful list!).

My diagnosis was a 2cm invasive carcinoma in the left breast located directly under the nipple. In some books, there would be a series of technical jargon from this point, but I believe the technical information can be covered in books by better authorities on the matter.

One of the best things Dr. B did for me was to take *"Breast Cancer Treatment Guidelines for Patients"*, a very informative publication by the American Cancer Society and the National Comprehensive Cancer Network, off the shelf and highlight everything pertinent in the book as we were discussing it. This was extremely helpful as the book contained a decision tree – the kind that says, "if this is the case, then here are your options – if this other is the case, then these are your options, etc." The technical information was something I could then read and re-read, look up, study, and understand when I was able to think clearer.

Not only did he "mark up" the book, but he also drew diagrams on flipcharts, in different colors for clearer explanation (little did I know then what kind of artist he was, but I found out later some of his true talents!)

There were a lot of choices thrown at me from lumpectomy to mastectomy to reconstruction (insert scream and pulling at hair image), and there were decisions that had to be made. My emotions were very high, but in the end I felt good (and still do to this day) about my decisions.

Basically, since the cancer was directly under my nipple, for me the decisions started with either a lumpectomy (or in this case, since the surgery would require me to lose the front part of the breast it was also known as a partial mastectomy) or a full mastectomy and whether I wanted reconstruction done. Dr. B explained that there weren't any guarantees that even if I had a total mastectomy (both breasts) that this would not mean the cancer could not come back over time. We had a long discussion about the options since my cancer was in the nipple area, and it was small enough at 2 cm, that I opted for the partial mastectomy, which is essentially the same as a lumpectomy except that I was actually losing a definitive part of the breast. I asked him that all important question, "If I were your mother…" He laughed and said I was way too young to be his mother, but If I were his sister or wife (shoot – he's married and has 4 kids – oh, well, he is still easy on the eyes!), yes, this would be the surgery he would recommend.

Okay, then. One of the things I really dislike in life is indecision. I don't always make the right decision, although I did in this matter, but being a "fence sitter" makes me crazy. I would rather make the decision and move on than sit there dangling my feet off the fence!

I believe that Dr. B is a fantastic doctor and I did and do trust him with my life. When I asked him once why he chose this particular focus, he told me that there was so much controversy in the field of breast cancer, and it was always changing with new updates in medicine. I think that is what keeps it interesting for him. When I was diagnosed, he told me there would be some decisions to make, and he could advise me, but only I could make the decisions. I know some people do not want this option, as they would rather just say to the doctor, "Do whatever you think is the best thing", and others who refuse to do anything and let nature take its course. If you have been reading this book from the beginning, you already know that I wanted all the information I could find so I could make a decision that I felt that I could live with.

Some of the decisions you face are what type of treatment you want, including how much of the breast you want removed, what type of follow-up you want after that, including reconstruction, removal of the lymph nodes, radiation, chemotherapy, and what type of long-term treatment you want, including medications like Tamoxifen or a variety of the newer drugs on the market. A lot of this decision is based on how quickly the cancer had been discovered, if there are other parts of your body affected by the cancer, and what your general health is at the time of the diagnosis, but we'll talk more about that in later chapters.

The surgery was scheduled for two weeks later and we were ready to go.

As I was leaving the office, I handed Dr. B, and his wonderful nurse, Nancy, each a big red foam clown nose – the first of many distributed along the path! I also left a nose for his staff person, Becky, who became my vital link to Dr. B. I think at that moment they felt they may not be dealing with their "normal" patient. And, I can tell you, I am described in many ways, with many adjectives, but "normal" is rarely one of them! I told them they were now officially part of my Humor Team, and we were getting on with it! Little did I know that the nose exchange would be the first of many "creative" episodes with Dr. B and his delightful nurse and staff!!

Lesson Five – *Recruit or "hire" (no cost involved) your personal Humor Team! Sometimes it is difficult to laugh at the situation, at other times, the only sense you can make out of life is a sense of humor. Other people can help you keep your spirits up and look for ways to see the lighter side of even the seemingly darkest situations.*

Chapter Five
Hiring the "H Team"!

"Among God's gifts to us are the people who love us."
— *Unknown Author*

For those of you reading this who know exactly what I am referring to, you are showing your age! For those of you who do not know the reference, there was a show on television called the "A Team" that ran from 1983 to 1987. Part of the introduction included, "If you have a problem, if no one else can help, and if you can find them, maybe you can hire the A-Team." The idea was to hire this group of wild outcasts from the military, who could do all kinds of things to find and take down the "bad guy". It was one of those shows where they could make explosives from a hairpin – you get the idea – very realistic! Hmmm, a group of wild outcasts, maybe that is a good definition of <u>my</u> "H Team"!!! (Just kidding team members, you really ARE the best!!!)

One of the most important things you can do for yourself and your recovery is to <u>Hire a Humor Team.</u> There is no cost involved for this team of supporters. No matter how "in control" of our lives we like to think we are, and trust me, I could be a poster child for independence, we truly should not face this alone. If you put your faith in God as I do, or other spiritual powers, be reminded that He is putting people on your path for a reason. For me, it was a team of people. I called them my own personal Humor Team. The team came complete with red clown noses, which is not a prerequisite, but it worked for me. I knew that when I was diagnosed, I was going to need people in my life who would make me laugh when I felt like crying, or laugh with me when I felt like celebrating, or to simply understand the quiet side of humor when I needed to be quiet.

As a professional clown, I already had a rather wild and unruly group of friends who regularly wore red clown noses and big funky shoes around me most of the time, so it wasn't really a huge stretch to hire them on for another "gig"; this was just a little different charge. Let me think about this, I am asking you to be goofy, supportive, and wild and crazy – you know your usual demeanor. In a later chapter I talk about "the wild party" which was a very special event, but throughout this journey, my Humor Team is what kept me going.

Members included my family and closest friends, so almost anything was accepted as part of the support system. It actually was a great lead into telling people what was going on. Conversations went a little like this, "Hi, Kathy, I just wanted to let you know that I have been diagnosed with breast cancer, and wanted to know if you would be on my Humor Team?" It seemed as though when I framed it in that manner, the severity of the cancer diagnosis was reduced both for me and the person I was talking to. I know this sounds a little strange, but that was the way it worked. This is another example of not being able to change things, but changing our own personal response.

The Humor Team was there for me every step of the journey in a lot of different ways. That was one of the neatest aspects of the team, there were so many different people and each person had their own idea of their responsibilities as a team member. One team member would send me a daily joke. Another member made a personal set of positive saying cards, each was individually wrapped in the bright colors that I love, and included the card and a bible verse. The idea was to keep these with me at all times, and when I needed an extra boost, I could pull a card out of my pocket and be refreshed. Other members sent me daily e-mails with crazy stories to make me laugh.

In fact, one member, a very well endowed member, went so far as to offer to donate some of that "endowment" for my reconstruction. Now that's a dedicated friend!

    There is another point about hiring or recruiting your Humor Team that is extremely important. When you receive this type of diagnosis, not only do you not know how to respond, but the people around you don't know how to respond either – it just catches you off guard. Although I had quite a few members of "my team" on board, and they understood what I was asking, there was still some trepidation on their part about the actual role. One day after I returned from the doctor, I e-mailed all of my team and told them I just wanted to "keep them <u>abreast</u>" of the situation! This simple play on words acted as a catalyst for the team to lighten up and laugh with me. One member of my team told me later that she wasn't really sure what she was supposed to do, but, when she read this message, she knew it was going to be okay to laugh, and from there the healing ball started to roll!

Criteria for Recruiting Your Humor Team

    As you are reading this information, you may be thinking about who you would ask to join your personal Humor Team. What does a Humor Team member have to do? Should they be comedians? Is it required that they are always laughing? The answer to these questions is a resounding "no". From my perspective, one of the main requirements of a Humor Team member is a firm belief that by looking for the lighter side of any situation, the healing process is faster and better. For some people this is an easy mission, but for others it takes a great deal of effort.

    My mother was probably one of the best examples of this transition. As a registered nurse, and my mother, she found absolutely no humor in her daughter being diagnosed with breast cancer. I go into a little more detail about this situation in the chapter on telling others, but the idea of any type of humor at this challenging time was very difficult for her. It wasn't until she was actually here with me and she met the members of the Humor Team that she gained a better insight into the great value they were playing in my recovery. (In fact, she was so fascinated by this whole concept of a Humor Team, that she later gave a speech about it to her local Toastmasters club.)

Please know that the Humor Team concept is not about laughing at an illness or tragic situation, but it is a way of providing a coping mechanism to make a choice about some things that you cannot control in your life. As I mentioned before, this type of diagnosis can put you into a true tail spin and everything around you feels like it is out of control. In many ways, you get a sense that your body has betrayed you and you need to find that sense of control somewhere, anywhere. Looking at how you respond to a difficult situation can offer some sense of that personal control.

Scientific Benefits of Laughter

The scientific benefits of a Humor Team are great. The effect of humor on healing has been studied for a while, but reseachers are just now starting to see the true benefits of humor and faith in the healing process. There are even programs now that are partnering people from science and religion to study faith and healing, and combining it with humor and healing.

In the late 1970's, Norman Cousins wrote a book titled, *Anatomy of an Illness: as Perceived by the Patient*, where he examined the healing power of humor and its effects on the body when dealing with an illness. Cousins' book actually prompted people in the medical field to take a closer look at the connection between laughter and the body's own ability to heal. More recently the benefits are being explored as people start "Laughter Clubs" around the globe. In fact, I mentioned this during one of my surgeries and the anesthesiologist told me his parents belonged to a laughter club in India and felt that the experience had changed their lives. Even in our clown group, we take time out for a belly laugh every time we get together. As with language, human beings are supposedly the only species capable of laughter. Laughter is actually a complex response that involves many of the same skills used in solving problems. My theory is that God must have given us this gift of laughter for a reason – and I say one reason is for healing the mind, heart, body, and soul!

There are quite a few pieces of research out there that suggest the ability to laugh is helpful to those coping with major illnesses and the stress of life's problems. Researchers are now saying laughter can do a lot more as it can basically bring balance to all the components of the immune system, which helps us fight off diseases. Laughter seems to reduce levels of certain stress hormones. Laughter also seems to provide a sort of safety valve that shuts off the flow of stress hormones and the fight-or-flight compounds that swing into action in our bodies when we experience stress, anger or hostility. These stress hormones suppress the immune system, increase the number of blood platelets (which can cause obstructions in arteries) and raise blood pressure. When we're laughing, natural killer cells that destroy tumors and viruses increase and help set the foundation for healing.

Laughter also increases the concentration of salivary immunoglobulin A, which defends against infectious organisms entering through the respiratory tract.

What may surprise you is the fact that researchers estimate that laughing 100 times is equal to 10 minutes on the rowing machine or 15 minutes on an exercise bike. Laughing can be a total body workout! Blood pressure is lowered, and there is an increase in vascular blood flow and in oxygenation of the blood, which further assists healing. Laughter also gives your diaphragm and abdominal, respiratory, facial, leg and back muscles a workout. That's why you often feel exhausted after a long bout of laughter — you've just had an aerobic workout! And, you know, it just feels GREAT!!! You may want to check out this rather unusual form of exercise. It really can make the difference in your life, too! You can learn more about laughter (and a lot of other things) and the actual process that takes place in your body as you laugh by checking out: www.howstuffworks.com.

My Humor Team took up the charge of laughter and certainly made the difference in my life and recovery!

Lesson Six – *Be prepared to put up your personal "shield of protection". When you share the news that you have breast cancer with people, you will discover that everyone has a sister, cousin, friend, or whomever who has been through this before. IF YOU feel like you want to talk to others about the experience that is fine. If you don't, politely tell them that you aren't ready for this right now, but you appreciate the offer. This is indeed YOUR diagnosis and life. YOU have to decide what you need and want. Don't be afraid to be polite and just say, "No, thank you, I don't want to talk with you about this right now." Build your own "shield of protection"!*

Chapter Six
The Waiting Days

"When you're down to nothing; God is up to something.
--Unknown Author

This chapter is more of a chronological account of the days leading up to the surgery. The chapter tends to jump around a bit due to the various ideas I wanted to convey, but then again, my life was jumping around a whole bunch and it was difficult to keep everything in order.

The days between the diagnosis and the actual surgery were filled with a roller coaster of emotions. The only time I had actually come close to crying was on the drive home from the surgical biopsy when I sat in the car, eyes dripping, trying to figure out how to tell my two daughters, then ages 17 and 20. Not only was it not the best news to tell them that their mother may have cancer, but now they may be at a greater risk for developing breast cancer in their lives.

My Mantra

One of the first things I did was to develop a mantra for myself. A mantra can be a word, phrase, song, whatever you choose that can help you fiercely fight any negative thoughts that come into your mind, and trust me, they will! Mine just came to me. If you remember as a child reciting Frere Jacques?, or Are You Sleeping?, or Where is Thumbkin?, then you get the tune. My variation went like this:

> I am healthy
> I am healthy
> Yes, I am
> Yes, I am
> Soft and pink and healthy
> Soft and pink and healthy
> Yes, I am
> Yes, I am

    The "I am healthy" and "Yes, I am" came very easily, but I had to really think hard for the "Soft and pink and healthy" part. This may sound minor, but it actually is a very important part of the song.

    I remembered reading a story once about positive thinking and visualization. This particular story was about a man who was diagnosed with cancer. He asked his doctor what cancer cells looked like and what healthy cells looked like. He then visualized constantly a waterfall of healthy cells falling onto his body washing the bad cells away until he was completely rid of the bad cells. In this story, the cancer disappeared and the man fully believed it was because of his visualization. Some may think this is ridiculous, and that is their opinion, but there is a great deal of research out there that looks at the power of the mind over the body for healing and performance. This is not just in cancer and illness recovery, but also in the world of sports, learning, and martial arts, just to name a few.

    For my song I had to decide what I visualized as a healthy breast. In my mind, a healthy breast was soft and pink. Dr. B told me the cancer tissues were hard, so obviously it had to be soft tissue, and pink is a warm, comforting color. Besides, it fit my song perfectly and stayed!! I had my mantra, and I certainly used this little healthy ditty to help with my healing!

    The day following the diagnosis went well. I was trying to come to terms with the diagnosis and thinking about how life was going to be a little different for the next few months.

I shared my mantra with my closest friends and after some uproarious belly laughing we agreed that at least I could whistle the tune and people would just think I was going back to my childhood and thinking about Frere Jacques!!

It took awhile for me to be able to say "I have breast cancer", but eventually I got to the point that I could stand up straight and say it clearly, certainly not as a matter of pride, but as a matter of fact. I had to accept the fact to be able to start the recovery.

Some nights I would go to bed with my mantra in my head over and over again. Other nights I envisioned a brightly colored kite that was sailing in the clouds. When I first started having this visualization, I found myself hanging onto the kite string. I would think, "God, I am sending all of my concerns and worries to you. Please take them." I would feel good for a second, but then I would yank that kite string right back down. I knew I was making progress when I could load my concerns and worries onto the kite and actually visualize letting go of the string for good. I had finally learned how to let go and let God take it! I remember reading somewhere that we should, "Give all your worries and concerns to God. He's going to be up all night anyway."

I also found a very brightly-colored collage that I adopted as one of my healing visualizations. It was actually a picture from an old calendar, but the bright colors made me happy when I looked at it. I started to visualize that my body was filled with all these brightly colored HEALTHY cells and there were no ugly color cells. Again, it may sound strange, but it worked or me. I even got Dr. B to "buy into it" and he told me how to see the healthy cells – round and almost plump.

The "Curse" of a Great Attitude

There was a strange phenomenon happening while I was at work during this time. I seem to have a reputation for being upbeat and projecting a positive attitude in most situations with my co-workers. As the news of my situation became more commonly known, I had an overwhelming feeling that I was "being watched". I certainly believe this feeling was self-imposed, but I had this tremendous sense that people were watching me to see how I would handle the situation. I knew in my heart that I was allowed to cry, be angry, laugh, or do whatever I needed to do to cope, but this overwhelming sense was instrumental in keeping my emotions in check. Overall, I think it was actually beneficial, because each time I felt like crying, I would think of the mantra and start feeling better from the inside out. I would start whistling again and the day just seemed brighter. This feeling of happiness and peace worked very well for me to help with the healing. Again, this is a personal diagnosis, and how you CHOOSE to respond is as individual as you are.

A Mixture of Strange Days

I had decided that maybe a few movies would take my mind off of things. The only stipulation was that I would only watch funny movies. I love funny movies and old television shows. Carol Burnett is one of my favorite actresses and her old shows were a fantastic addition to my Healing Library. We went out and rented "The Crew" which is like a mobster version of Grumpy Old Men. It has some very funny scenes and ideas to offer, and most importantly, no tear-jerking scenes. Well, that is probably the case for people who have not just been diagnosed with breast cancer! As it turned out, the last scene was a very touching (and brief, I mean very brief – like one minute) moment with a father and daughter. The tears started and I had a feeling the floodgates had just opened. I mentioned to CJ that I thought I was going to cry for a little while. The next 45 minutes was spent in the bathroom crying uncontrollably.

From there I calmed down and moved to the bedroom. After a few minutes of quiet, the gates opened again and I continued to cry.

I had been lying awake at night and thinking of the many things yet to do, but this night was the first night I REALLY cried for a very long time - I mean long as in the length of time I cried. I got to the end of the tissue box and said, "Well, I guess that is enough crying - I am out of tissues."

While I was calming down, I picked up the water bottle I usually have beside my bed. As I was taking long, slow drinks, it dawned on me that I had never really mastered the art of blowing across the water bottle and achieving melodious tunes (a breast cancer diagnosis can do strange things to the mind!). Thinking there was no time like the present, I started with small sounds as I was trying to position the air stream just right. After I caught on a little better, I moved up to a Jingle Bells masterpiece on the water bottle. My faithful (actually only faithful as long as I have the food in my hands, or am the only one left in bed in the morning!) companion, Tigger (a Lhasa Apso breed dog), was on the bed. I am not sure what it sounded like to him (you know, there is a critic in every crowd) but he started yelping and growling, then he jumped off the bed and raced down the hall, and back and forth. He must have kept this up for at least 15 minutes. The crying that had taken most of my immediate energy soon gave way to a deep, hilarious laughter that continued for the entire 15 minutes — what a wonderful quick change in emotions. Instead of feeling spent from the crying, I actually went to bed energized and feeling very good.

There were a few days that I had trouble sleeping. I don't really think I was overly worried or concerned, but my mind just wandered all over the place. The one and only thing that helped calm me down was my little "I am healthy" song. I know I must have sung it to myself at least fifty times and fell asleep with it in my head. Although this may sound minor, you have to find something that works for YOU! If you are truly dedicated to trying to find and celebrate the lighter side of recovery, you have to be willing to step outside your comfort zone. And, yes, sometimes your sanity zone to try something that may seem strange, but can calm your mind.

    I had thought of more questions to ask Dr. B, and he had told me to e-mail him if I with any additional questions. This was before the new HIPPA (Health Insurance Portability and Accountability Act – basically patient privacy issues) regulations, and quite frankly, it was certainly better for me from a patient's perspective to be able to contact the doctor. I had forgotten to ask about the type of anesthetic that I would have for the surgery, and a couple of other minor thoughts, so I sent him a quick message.

    When I received his reply to the e-mail, I was in a small panic. He told me the type of anesthetic should be an epidural (in the most simplistic terms, a needle stuck in your back near the spine). He liked this type of anesthetic because he thought it would be much better for me than general anesthetic. What he didn't know was that I was terrified by the mere thought of an epidural. I am sure it goes back to my days of having children when they talked about an epidural having so many side effects. Obviously, medicine had come a long way in twenty years, but I was still very concerned.

    I went to the internet and did a couple of searches to see what to expect. Although the internet is an extremely valuable informational tool, be aware of this method of research. There is a fine line between gathering information to make decisions, and getting information that may scare you. One of the first sites I searched was about the benefits AND risks of this procedure. If I was afraid before, I really panicked after reading this information. I quickly exited the site and sat in my chair concerned. I know how very important the mental attitude is, so I forced myself to go back to the site and read only the benefits. I found one I really liked (faster recovery time from the anesthetic), thought about that for a minute, and then quickly exited the site.

Please understand, it is very important to gather the information necessary to make an informed decision, but when planting subconscious thoughts, the negative thoughts are the most harmful. I needed to take that positive thought and hold it in place until I spoke to the anesthesiologist about the issue. The internet is one source of information, but a real live person is another and he or she can respond directly to all the questions that I needed to ask about what would happen to me personally.

A Series of "Days"

Much like the different stages of mourning, or depression, I had different stages of "dealing". What I discovered was that I had "days". For example, I had my "Mad Day". I was driving home from presenting a workshop two days after my biopsy. My thoughts drifted to, "Why am I going through this? I know people who smoke and drink and do drugs, and THEY don't have breast cancer!" I was just angry at this happening to me.

Then there was my "Panic Day". It went something like this. Conversation to myself – "Dr. B said we can wait two weeks because two weeks won't make a difference, but how does he really know? Obviously, this wasn't on the mammogram last year and now it is at 2 cm. He said the average size is 1½ cm. If this is already bigger than the average, how does he know it won't grow and take over my whole breast before the surgery? And, actually, since the biopsy was on the 8th and the surgery isn't until the 25th that is almost three weeks. What if the pathology report is wrong? What if he goes in on the 25th and this thing has grown and now I don't have a choice? What if it is really aggressive, and exactly what are these cells doing in there in my breast? I am sure they aren't sleeping. What if it is like a Pac-Man game and the bad cells are just eating away at the good cells, and what if..."? Oh, yes, and then I took a breath!!

The mantra was getting a workout, and I was even getting good at putting some hip action into it and singing it with gusto, usually in the car or privacy of my own home, but not always. There were a few times I got caught in the hallway at work whistling and dancing to this strange little ditty.

This period also had days of celebration. One of the first things that may be checked when you are diagnosed is a chest X-ray and blood work. Dr. B ordered these for me immediately after discussing the diagnosis. I called Dr. B's office to see if they had the results of the blood work. Since this was the second of the two tests (the chest X-ray was the first and that was clear of cancer indicators) it was important in my mind to find some positives while I was waiting. The nurse reported that the blood tests all came back clear – woo-hoo!!! Two tests showing no clear spread of cancer anywhere else!!! Where's the champagne and hot fudge sundaes???

Starting to Say Good-Bye

I also wanted to know about removing the bandage from the biopsy. To some people this may sound absolutely crazy, but others will understand exactly what I am about to say. I needed time to say good-bye to my nipple and areola (the area around the nipple), a new word that I think I could have gone through my whole life not knowing what it meant. Now I was going to be losing mine, a part of me that I had for 42 years, and I needed to say good-bye.

During my first meeting with Dr. B, he told me that surgeons no longer go in for exploratory biopsy surgery and just take the woman's breast if it turns out to be cancer. This was the method followed by many in the healthcare profession not that many years ago. The woman would have no idea what to expect when she awoke in recovery, whether or not she would have a breast or breasts. He said he had never done this type of radical surgery without the woman fully knowing what to expect, and, thankfully, it is not a common practice any more.

I think the closure part of losing a breast is very important to the healing process. One of the regrets I have is that I didn't get a picture of my breast before I went into the hospital the first time. After that first surgery, the breast wasn't exactly the same. It still looked healthy, but the stitches were showing and it just didn't look the same. I think about what these women would have gone through when they went into the operating room with a full breast and came out not knowing what they were going to find. There is a great value in closure and, thankfully, more modern medicine.

Anyway, back to the story. My breast was covered with a square, clear piece of plastic skin-like tape with green edges. CJ mentioned that it looked like a flag from a foreign country. Under the tape was a piece of gauze over the nipple about the size of a silver dollar. I could not see the nipple and I wanted to see it before it was gone. I called Dr. B's office and asked the nurse if Dr. B would leave the bandage on until the surgery. She responded yes, as long as it didn't get wet. I asked the nurse what I should do if it got wet. She said that the incision was stitched and should be healing at this point (over a week after the surgery) so it should be fine if the bandage fell off. Just be sure the stitches do not come out. Okay, I had my plan. Tonight I would peel a small edge from the side of the tape and shower in the morning. If the bandage happened to get wet, I had better take it off! Note: I do not recommend that YOU do this, I just had to see Inny for a while before she was gone, and I would NOT have even considered proccediny if the nurse said it would damage my breast – you know the one that was going to be disfigured in nine days!! Okay, okay, so maybe I would have anyway. After all, what did I have to lose – this part of the breast was going anyway!

Before I did anything, I asked CJ to take a picture. For me it was important to have pictures of the different stages so I could look back ten years from now and see how far I have come. This was looking for the future reasons to celebrate. By now you have probably already decided that I am always looking for a reason for a party!!

I started slowly and just peeled off a little edge, then down horizontally and cut it down to size. At least it was smaller. This would be enough for now.

Preparing For the Surgery – Hospital Style

As part of the preparation for surgery at our hospital, I was asked to see the nurse and anesthesiologist at the hospital as part of the pre-op information. They wanted to go over my complete medical history to make sure there weren't any surprises, on either side, on the day of the surgery. There were certainly a couple of funny things that happened during this meeting!

First, the nurse went over the medical history form I filled out regarding past illnesses and other things they needed to know before doing the surgery. She made the usual statements, "No history of heart problem, no diabetes, etc., etc. It looks like you are in good health." I couldn't help but crack up laughing and said to her, "Yeah, great health except that I have cancer!" I don't think she realized what she had said and a smile crept across her face. Her next question absolutely floored me. She asked, "Have you had any major traumas in your life in the last year, like relationship, job change, or health issues?" (Yes, she actually said this!) I looked at her and said, "No (with a long pause), except for this cancer thing!" I was concerned she was going to toss me out of the room, but again she just smiled and went on with the paperwork. I think I have discovered that this diagnosis has sharpened my ability to laugh at some of the craziest things. This is indeed a good thing. Since I cannot change it, looking for the funniest things or lighter things happening around me became the fabric of life that I was holding on to.

The nurse continued to go over the information and told me what I could expect when I arrived at the hospital. She told me what would happen in the Nuclear Medicine department in regards to injecting a blue dye needed to locate the sentinel lymph node (which I explain in greater detail in a later section) and what I should expect from recovery. She was very good at expressing that this was general information, and that everyone responds differently. This is excellent advice for anyone dealing with an illness, both for the good and the bad. Just because someone else experienced pain or problems, does not mean you will! The importance of this realization is that sometimes we set our minds up to expect pain or discomfort and we psychologically feel it because we mentally "expect" to.

Next, I was to speak to the anesthesiologist. I was anxious to discuss the epidural procedure recommended by Dr. B. I expressed my concern and he went over the procedure. I was still feeling a bit anxious, but felt I was wasting his time with frivolous concerns. Finally, I said, "Listen, I know this may seem minor to you, but I am REALLY concerned. Can you tell me exactly what will happen?" He sat back and took me through every step of the procedure. He told me that I would have an I.V. sedation so I wouldn't feel a thing. Then the epidural needle would be placed between my shoulder blades and a tube (called a catherization procedure) would be inserted to provide a place for the needle to administer the drugs. He said when the surgery was complete, they would pull out the catherization and I would not feel any of the actual procedure. His professional and caring manner really put me at ease. Throughout the whole conversation he mentioned, "Remember, this is your choice. We can do whatever you feel comfortable with." (This is a very important point. Much of what was happening to me was MY choice. The professionals were giving me the options and I was able to choose from my comfort level.)

I had experienced pain in my shoulder blades for a couple of years from a previous fall. I was concerned that this might make that worse, so I turned that negative thought into a positive one and told myself, maybe, just maybe I would wake from the surgery and the epidural would have actually acted as acupuncture and taken away the pain I was experiencing! I do not want you to think that I was spending my time lying to myself about what was going to happen. Since I truly did not know what was going to happen, as far as how I would respond, again it was more beneficial to plant the positive thought seed, than to dwell on the negative.

I told the anesthesiologist that I had 100% confidence in Dr. B, and he (the anesthesiologist) was the expert in his field, at least compared to me, so I felt it was my best choice to go with what they were recommending. I reminded myself that Dr B. had performed hundreds of operations and that was a pretty large study group to decide that his patients had a better response from epidurals. If that was good enough for him, it was good enough for me, again, reinforcing the importance of the relationship YOU establish with your health care providers.

I left the meeting feeling more relaxed about the upcoming operation.

Staying Busy

The operation was still eight days away and I had to keep myself occupied. For me personally, if I sat around the house worrying, I would have a much more difficult time with the surgery than if I kept moving. (This is a personal choice. If you don't have a lot to keep you busy, I would suggest starting a project of some type. It could be starting a book you have always wanted to read (OR WRITE!), a cross-stitch piece, or maybe a journal of your experiences. Personally, I feel it is best to have a project that you can "complete". This gives you a sense of accomplishments, and right now you need to be celebrating even the smallest accomplishments in your life!)

Back to Saying Good-Bye

I finally decided the bandage was going!! Not only did I need to start the visual good-bye process, but I also was concerned about the skin beneath the bandage. If it was going to be covered for 2 ½ weeks, and then another one put on from the next surgery, I wanted it to be able to breathe a bit. I discovered as I peeled the bandage off that the skin-like tape was actually very soft and the skin under the breast was not chapped except in a couple of small places.

I thought about why I was upset about losing the nipple and realized the "good-bye" process was due, in large part, to this being a part of my body for so long, not only in the length of time I had spent with this perky little part, but that it was a part of my life that would never be the same. I used this nipple (and the other one!) to nurse my two beautiful daughters as they began their lives. One of these nipples was going to be removed and replaced by a scar. I wasn't concerned at all that the scar would be ugly or gross looking, but that it would be an indicator of a permanent, physical change to my body. I just needed to say thank you and good-bye.

When I took the bandage off, the tip of the nipple was dry and raw from lack of lotion and the usual tender loving care of the shower. It still felt good to feel and touch the nipple. The thought of it being gone forever in a week brought tears to my eyes. I was thankful that this didn't have to be a total mastectomy, but there was going to be a major, lifelong difference in the shape of my breasts, and I was sure there would be psychological issues to deal with immediately after the surgery.

One of the stranger things I noticed was that the breast under the nipple was numb. I hadn't noticed this until I touched the skin and realized I couldn't feel the touch. Had I not been going in the following week for surgery, I would have called Dr. B's office to see what was going on. I couldn't recall reading or seeing anything about my breast being numb ten days after surgery. If I was not going to require additional surgery, I would have called right away, just to set my mind at ease but, instead, I just wrote it down on the list of questions I had beside my bed to ask Dr. B on Thursday before the surgery. I also wanted to mention to Dr. B that he should remember to tell his patients that there may be a change in sensation for quite a while. So many times we are too close to the situation, and forget what it is like when someone experiences something for the first time. A good doctor learns from his or her patients, too!

A Rather Strange but Funny Day!

Then there was my "Funny Day" where everything I thought about was funny, or I could put a funny twist on it. I started the morning with a 20 second belly laugh. Yes, I know it sounds crazy, but as I mentioned before, there is a lot of research indicating how laughing can help make the body heal. The belly laugh is really a very simple exercise and can be done alone or in the company of others, but you might want to make sure there aren't any people in the group looking for that "extra reason" to have you institutionalized – this might just do it!

All you do is START LAUGHING and continue for 20 seconds. When you try this for the first time, it might help to look at something funny. For example my dog, Tigger, usually helps me with the goofy expressions on his face, or I think of something that has happened in my life that was especially funny. Although I know this may sound a little on the loony side, you will be amazed at how this helps to loosen your body and reminds you HOW to laugh, in case you have forgotten! In fact, there is research that provides strong indications that your body doesn't even know if you are sincerely laughing or just faking it – the results are the same!

From there it just seemed like everything took on a humorous life of its own. Before you continue reading, remember that people handle a cancer diagnosis in a variety of ways. The purpose of this book is to look at all of the emotions that go with a diagnosis, but especially looking for and celebrating the lighter side on the path to recovery.

I realized that the day was going to be a bit different when I was walking into work with a co-worker. We exchanged the usual pleasantries; you know the, "Good Morning. How are you today?" I was SOOOO close to saying, "Hey, I am just great today, well, except for this cancer thing." (This co-worker knew nothing about my diagnosis and I wasn't prepared to share it with her at this particular moment.) Just the thought of what I actually almost said struck a funny bone and I just started to laugh inside. Then it got even worse!!

As you may recall, all of this happened in my life just a month after the 9/11 terrorist attacks on New York and Washington, DC. Everyone was edgy about the continued threats, the anthrax scare, and everything going on in the world at that time. My co-worker continued to ask me if I had heard about the scare at the Three Mile Island Nuclear plant the previous night. Apparently, there was a threat and they closed the airports, etc. I had not heard this news, but (again, this was funny emotion invading my brain!!) all I could think of was, "Hey, this is great, I won't be going through this radiation thing alone. Three Mile Island goes; the whole community will be going with me. I will have all kinds of company."

Please, <u>please</u> do not think this is morbid. Of course I would never want to experience or have others experience the threat of a nuclear attack, but it was a way of releasing the stress and anxiety about having cancer. Stress and anxiety can affect you in so many different ways, and everyone is completely different. That, too, is a reason to celebrate. There really aren't any set rules on how we MUST deal with this or any other difficult situation. It was another choice I was making – to look for the lighter side, WHEREVER I could find it, and celebrate!

Later in the morning I was walking downtown with a friend who did know about the cancer. As we met, she said, "So how are you doing today?" This time it was just too much. I very quickly replied, "I'm feeling great today, except for this cancer thing!" We both laughed and laughed simply about the idea. After I told her about my experience with the nurse at the hospital the day before, we laughed some more! It feels so good to laugh!

During this time, my Humor Team was really taking up the job! I was bombarded with goofy e-mails, funny jokes, messages at my desk, and just about anything else they could conjure up in their zany little brains!

Waiting and Waiting

There was still a week before the major surgery – almost a milepost day, and I was reflecting, between the laughing, about why this all seemed so bizarre. Finally it dawned on me. Of course this was bizarre or weird or surreal as I came to call it shortly after the diagnosis – I couldn't have cancer – I felt fine!!! The thought of taking my seemingly healthy body into the hospital in just one week to lose part of my breast and start radiation, possibly medication for the next five years, and chemotherapy where I may lose my hair, possibly feeling sick and fatigued just did not make any sense. I FELT FINE!!! This is one of the dangers of cancer. We feel fine so when we have to go in for a check-up or should go in because we discover a change, whether it be the breast or elsewhere, we hesitate and tell ourselves it can't be cancer, I FEEL FINE!

I was really on a roll today. I was telling a friend about the diagnosis and it dawned on me…Who said I had to have a straight incision? Dr. B was great at giving me a lot of options; I thought I might as well ask him about one more. I firmly believe that the answer to anything is always "no" if you don't ask, so I was going to ask! Many people had told me what a wonderful surgeon he was, so I thought my next e-mail would not be an especially difficult request.

I sent an e-mail message to Dr. B and asked him if it was possible for him to make the incision in the shape of a smile instead of straight across. My theory was that I could have two eyes later tattooed or put on by the permanent markers they use in radiation or chemotherapy and at least when I looked in the mirror, my newly formed breast would be smiling back at me! Actually, I started the message by saying that "Now you probably already think I am a little "touched", but I have been thinking a great deal about reconstruction options and I have a serious request to make". I thought, "If he doesn't have me committed after the surgery, I will be surprised!" He actually wrote back that we would see what he could do, but couldn't make any promises – I bet that request made for some interesting conversation in the Doctor's lounge!

With less than a week to go, it seemed as though my thoughts were all over the place. There were moments of calm, never real relaxation but at least calming, where I realized that by this time next week, the cancer would be out of my body. Of course, the nipple goes with it, but I was trying to mentally prepare for that part of the recovery. I think I felt as though I had a better chance somehow because of the faith I had in Dr. B. I knew that God would be working through his hands, and that I truly was going to be fine.

Another Major Step

My youngest daughter, Lacey, was attending a 20 week program in a city about 90 miles from our house. We made the trek every other Saturday, and this was the day. It was just the two of us on the ride and it gave us a nice opportunity to talk about her feelings and my feelings as the week of surgery approached. One thing I can't emphasize enough is that you must have an open line of communication with your closest family members. After I told her the true prognosis, she asked some questions, and in the same way I continually thought of questions to ask Dr. B, she also thought of additional questions as the time went by. This day we joked about wigs that I may need, hats, and how her life was impacted by the diagnosis. We discussed when she should get her first mammogram, and how we both TRULY felt about what was happening. The talk was good and necessary for both of us.

Another funny thought came to me as we were traveling to her class. When I was pregnant with her, my second child, over seventeen years ago, I was very sick. During my first pregnancy I experienced morning sickness for the first three months and then on what seemed like the 91^{st,} day it stopped and I felt fine through the delivery. However, my second pregnancy was very different! With this one, I think I started to throw up the very first day of conception and didn't stop until after she was delivered!! In fact, I wound up in the hospital for a couple days when I was 3 or 4 months pregnant from dehydration. The reason this memory was so funny at the present time was because I mentioned to Lacey that, although I was worried about having to go through chemo, being pregnant with her certainly had prepared me if I was going to get sick from the chemo. I figured at the worse with chemo, even if I got sick every single day, which was unlikely, I still wouldn't be as sick as I was during my pregnancy with her, and look what a beautiful child came out of that mess! We truly laughed about the thought of chemo preparation, not that it was funny under normal circumstances, but you know, breast cancer is not a normal circumstance. Sometimes life has a way of throwing you a curveball!

After I dropped her off for her class, I had seven hours to roam around and find something to do. In the past, I had used this opportunity to shop or read, or find new places to explore. As I was driving down the highway, for some unknown reason my mind went back to just a few months before (June 2001) and the Relay for Life held in our area. If you are not familiar with this event, it is a 24 hour walk (around a track at a local high school) to raise money and awareness for the American Cancer Society. The company I work for usually has a number of people who walk in support of the program. This past year I was on one of the teams. What dawned on me is how I could have possibly known that in less than a year I would be a breast cancer survivor. The amazing thing about the day was the realization that this was the first time I thought of myself as a "survivor". No, it isn't that I thought I was going to die, in fact that thought never really crossed my mind. If circumstances would have been different, I am sure I may have gravitated to those thoughts. In reality I truly believed we had caught it early and that I had an excellent chance of full recovery. Recovery I had thought of before, but not the term "survivor". For some reason, on this day the thoughts were of being a survivor, not just any survivor, but a breast cancer survivor. It was oddly getting easier to not only say the words, "I have breast cancer", but to really understand what all that entailed and that I could indeed add the statement, "I am a breast cancer survivor" to my vocabulary. I firmly believe that this was another <u>major step in my recovery</u>.

    For many nights I had been reading a wonderful book before I went to bed (Norman Vincent Peale's, *In God We Trust*) and it had a soothing effect on my attitude and nerves. I truly wasn't concerned about the upcoming procedure and treatment. I knew it was going to mean a lot of changes, but that I would really be fine – I was diligently working on the "right" attitude to deal with the situation.

    When I awoke, I had two very quick thoughts. Looking back I think they were related for a distinct reason. The first thought was about reconstruction. Since my cancer was directly under the nipple, and Dr. B mentioned having reconstructive surgery at the time of the lumpectomy, could they really reattach my own nipple? I hadn't specifically asked that question. My mind started racing. (Keep in mind; this is three days before the surgery.) The questions went something like this — If I go to the computer quickly and e-mailed him, could it be worked out? Could they re-attach my own nipple? He said I could have met with a plastic surgeon last week and maybe we could have arranged the reconstruction at the same time. These questions were at such a furious pace that I broke out in a sweat! I had to check this out quickly.

To calm myself, I stated my little mantra song, "I am healthy…." However, for some reason, when I got to the "Soft and pink, and healthy" part, healthy is not what came out. My mind had changed it to "Soft and pink and <u>sexy!</u>" I stopped for a moment and reflected on the lyric change and, in all honestly, I think THAT was the start of the <u>self-image healing</u>. I had been spending so much time thinking about the physical change of losing my nipple and perhaps, subconsciously thinking about losing my sexuality with the nipple. This was the start of that healing process, and the mantra song changed.

By the way, I mentioned the "put my own nipple back on" thing to CJ and Mary. Both said they remembered Dr. B saying that, unfortunately, the cancer was so close to my nipple that he would be concerned about re-attaching it. And, after I thought about it, I think that if I had tried to pursue it and the cancer came back, I would always wonder if I had made the wrong decision.

Lesson Seven - Start and keep a "Recovery Folder", "Jolly Journal", "Humor File", or whatever you want to call it. This is a file to put things like the little notes from friends, cards that you receive, cartoons, or any other momento to look at in the future. There may be times when you are feeling low. When that is the case, pick up your folder and remind yourself of the many people who care, and what a difference you make in their lives.

Chapter Seven
A Truly WILD Party!!

"Laughter is the shortest distance between two people."
-- *Victor Borge*

There is a song that starts with "Oh, what a night", well this was definitely a night that I will always remember, for the rest of my life!!!

First, some of my Humor Team members and I attended a presentation at the local hospital. When I arrived, one of my Humor Team members, Anita, was already seated and ready for action. On her head she wore a beautiful felt striped hat, similar to a character from Dr. Seuss. She had a variety of beautiful hats waiting for all of the team members attending the presentation. Each hat was bright and colorful, either felt stripes or multi-colored sequins, and each was adorned with a white band that said "Tammy's Team", with a pink breast cancer awareness symbol in the middle. Mine was slightly differently in that it had multi-colored squares and each square had the name of a member of my Humor Team written in it. What a wonderful way to start the evening, but it just got better and better from there!

The presentation topic was "Positive Attitude: Improving Treatment Outcomes." Dr. Dean Schrock, author of *Doctors Orders: Go Fishing*, believes that a positive attitude can improve the recovery time for people with a serious illness. He also is convinced that when people have a greater "will to live" it can affect a patient's quality of life. Dr. Schrock gave an interesting presentation for about 1½ hours. It was great to hear a professional reinforce the philosophy that what I was trying to do with my recovery team, by using humor and a positive attitude was actually proven in research to make a difference. I know it was making a difference in my life!!

After the presentation, it was time for a party. When all of this first started happening, I said to my dear friend, Linda, that I think I needed a party. Linda is never one to turn down that challenge, and she and the other dear members of my Humor Team got together and gave me a party that I will never forget!! More about that in a minute...

One of the things I have discovered through all of this is that people around you take their cues from YOU, not just when it comes to a serious illness, but also in response to a lot of different situations in life. Don't ever think as you are reading this book that I do not believe breast cancer is a serious illness. I most certainly do, and it was happening to me. I have already mentioned a number of times that I could not change the diagnosis, only the way I responded to the diagnosis. The combination of verbal and non-verbal cues is very powerful in communication, and especially when the subject matter at hand is very serious. I talk about that a little more in the section on how to tell others.

When all of this started happening, and I talked to my closest friends, I was actually giving them permission to feel for what I was going through. As I mentioned before, with Linda, it was when I told her I wanted to keep her "abreast!" of the situation, that we both laughed, and that gave her permission to laugh with me. This was a very serious situation, and she didn't know how to respond until I let her see that I really was going to be okay, and the best way for me to get through this was with love and laughter.

Now, onto the party... It started as a "Keeping Abreast" party, but I was going through a lot of emotions associated with losing my nipple, so we decided to change the name of the party to a "Nipple Send Off" party. In the most simplistic terms, it was like a bachelorette party, with a few more pink breasts on the table! We all arrived after the presentation and the first thing I saw when I got there was a breast cake! Dottie had make an angel food (what else would you expect) cake mix into the shape of two breasts, complete with pink icing, and white "hugs" candy (similar to Hershey kisses, but white chocolate) with pink tips for the nipples. There were also a lot of spare candy "nipples" around the table, in case I needed to take a few on the day of surgery. The food also included pasta salad made with "Boob-shaped" (hey, that's what it said on the box!) pasta, vanilla wafers put together with icing tops and icing nipples in individual paper holders (two on a plate, of course!), and the usual party food. And, of course rolls of Lifesavers for all attendees!! This group was truly part of saving my life!

For this event, the Humor Team members were Linda, Jerry, Charlie, Mary, Anita, Dottie, and Marcy. "What a team" is right. I won't bore you with all the details, just a few highlights. The games we played included pin the pasties on the breasts (blindfolded using foam flowers, each adorned with a gold tassel); breast balloon pop (the skin tone balloons each had a pink areola of pink marker, and a nipple painted on with black, we closed our eyes and had to pop the balloons with a pin); and a heart search (Linda had placed 50 heart stickers of various sizes everywhere and we had to see who could find the most hearts). But, games were just a part of the festivities. My team wrote a song titled "Tammy" in my honor and sang it to the tune of "Mother" (T is for the terrific, etc…) complete with large letters and a true test in spelling. And, then onto the animals!! Each member donned an animal nose (walrus, pig (although he said it was a cow!), eagle, mouse, tiger, smile face, and dog (Dottie was on the toy guitar as the musical accompanist), and they sang my very own song – "Young McTammy Had A Farm", complete with all of the animal noises!!!

I won the heart game, and for the prize they gave me a box marked "Spare Parts Kit". Inside, Dottie had taken two plungers, filled the bottom with pillow stuffing and put plastic caps on for the nipples. She then put them in a beautiful lacy bra size 44 D (I don't want to reveal too much, but, personally, I have never made it that far in the alphabet, or that high numerically!! In fact, some might consider me one of the ol' "pirate's delight" – you know, the sunken chest!! I don't think it is THAT bad, but I am sure the only 44 I will ever see will be an age!!!).

Other highlights included a ton of crazy breast puns (not to be confused with breast pumps!), and a poster I hung in my office of two owls (Anita loves bird-watching). You know — two owls who "hoot" – a pair of hooters!! That gives you an idea of the flavor of the party.

For any of you who might think this is really distasteful, let me tell you how much we laughed. For over 2 hours, we laughed and laughed. In fact, I laughed so much I hurt the next morning, but it was a good hurt. I am so very thankful for my wonderful group of friends and their love. Their infectious attitude, love, and laughter made me realize that everything I would be facing over the next several months would work out fine.

For the last 20 minutes of the party we just sat and talked. They wanted to know what I needed at that moment. The team wanted to go to the hospital to be with me on the day of surgery and wanted to know what I would like them to do – sit with my family, tell jokes, whatever I wanted they wanted to do for me. I hand chose each of these people for the very special personality each one possessed. What we shared collectively was the love of laughter, knowing the value that humor plays in health care, and a mutual respect and compassion for one another. As you are choosing your team, keep all of these factors in mind.

Party Leftovers

One might wonder what you do with party leftovers from this type of party. Okay, okay, I had never had this type of party before, so I was new at this idea, but the answer seemed to come so easily. What does one do with a leftover breast cake – well, if one is going to have part of a breast removed by a top-notch doctor, then maybe he could use some spare parts! You got it, the leftover breast cake and several nipples found their way to Dr. B and his staff.

I dropped the boxed-up extra cake and nipples off to Dr. B's office in the box that read "spare parts" and with a note that read, "Hi Doc, I thought you might need some extra parts for my surgery on Thursday. I have also included some extra nipples, just in case." Actually, as I reflect back on this whole party and "gift" to Dr. B, I still laugh at the thought of this unusual gift. I wonder how many breast cakes he has received at his office???

This laughter stuff is so good for the soul, and sharing it with special people is truly a blessing!

Lesson Eight *– Find love and laughter everywhere. The world is filled with wonderful people and happy events. When we are facing something that is bigger than we are, a place where we feel we have lost control, it can be the love of our family and friends and the special moments sharing smiles and laughter that can change a dreary day into a meaningful and memorable moment. Being grateful for the people around you can give you strength and help support not only you, but also these important people in your life.*

Chapter Eight
Pennies from Heaven
(Or, a Wonderful Walk to the Wok)

"Friends are angels who lift us to our feet when our wings have trouble remembering how to fly."
— Unknown Author

I have spent a great deal of time talking about my Humor Team, and the world of difference they made in my life and recovery. Seven of the members of my humor team were also involved in another group called the Empowering Women. The eight of us all work at the same place and we formed the group as a way to support each other outside of the workplace.

In my job, I would go to many different offices and talked to a variety of people. When the conversation went momentarily to social issues I started to realize that I was hearing the same thing from a couple of different people. For example, one woman had a sweet, loving teenage son and thought that perhaps he had been abducted by aliens and replaced with this person who was suddenly unresponsive, didn't want to do homework, and was starting to rebel. I would talk with another woman and she told me a similar story – aliens again, and where was her sweet, loving son – surely this was not the child she gave birth to fourteen years ago! What I started to realize is that we all had similar problems, but we didn't know it. We thought we were alone in the challenges we were facing each day. After this went on for a few months, I talked with each of them and we decided to get together once a month and talk about our challenges, goals, dreams, etc. and basically form a support group. We had the added benefit that we all worked in the same place so that if work was an issue, we had a better understanding of the situation. We shared little gifts for birthdays, holidays, and when two women left to go to other jobs, we celebrated their new future.

The place we generally met for lunch was a outstanding local Chinese restaurant called the Golden Wok. The food is great, service is good, the owners are very cordial, and it is relatively close to the office. We all walked to the Wok (try to say that fast 10 times!!), and on our many walks, I would occasionally find a penny on the ground. I played around that if it was heads up, I would have good luck, and if it was tails up, I would give it to the first person I saw and we would both have good luck. Somewhere along the way I read about someone else doing this, but they said they picked up every penny they saw because our money reads, "In God We Trust", and the penny reminded them to trust in God no matter when or where they were.

Shortly before my surgery we decided to meet for our monthly visit. The rest of the Empowering Women decided it was going to be a party for me to celebrate life. It is hard to hide a gift bag when you are walking beside someone, so I picked up on the surprise rather easily – I'm quick that way! It took me a little while longer to realize the depth of the planning that went into this little gathering though.

It started as we were walking down the hallway just outside of my office. I looked down and there was a penny. I stopped and picked it up. I went a few more steps and there was another one, then another and twenty feet further another. I was really excited and figured someone had lost change out of his or her pockets. We were all chatting and laughing, as we usually do, and I was picking up pennies. There were seven between my office door and the door going outside. The strange thing was that when I went out the door, there was another penny. I started to think this was really odd, but it still did not dawn on me what was happening.

To get to the Wok, we come out a door and down a steep driveway, across a very, very busy intersection and down the street. All the way down the driveway there were pennies!!!! In fact, as we crossed the street there were more pennies – some even stuck in the hot tar on the road (I left those there!)! It took me until we came down the driveway and across the street to realize that I had been "had" – my fellow women had "planted" the pennies for me to find. The pennies lined the walkway up to the restaurant and when we got to the table, Mary had arranged for pennies to be set at everyone's place setting. The staff was really curious as to what was going on, but how do you explain to servers that you are a bunch of crazy women celebrating the loss of a nipple – it just doesn't come across very well!!

We were shown to our usual large round table in the back of the restaurant. It is great for a lot of reasons. It is at the back and we can giggle and laugh with each other without disturbing too many people. There was another reason I was glad to have the table on this particular day. Each person presented me with wonderfully thoughtful gifts for the occasion, including a beautiful plaque with the Serenity Prayer (a coincidence – I don't think so!), and a Speedy Gonzales Pez dispenser.

We had a wonderful lunch, and the love of this group of women was so powerful, that as much as I tried not to do it in public, I cried and cried as they all gave me little momento gifts, all covered with well wishes.

The people at the Wok were so accommodating to the pennies spread out all over and the crazy group of women. Although they didn't know what we were up to, I thank them for their gracious understanding – it truly was another special gathering!

Lesson Nine – Tell your closest family and friends in person, whenever possible. If you have chosen to take the positive approach, they will be better able to read your eyes, face, and body gestures to draw strength and forge on with you on the positive side of the path.

Chapter Nine
How to Tell Others

"I know God will not give me more than I can handle. I just wish He didn't trust me so much."
— *Mother Teresa*

Telling others took on a whole life by itself. As I mentioned before, my biggest concern was talking to my daughters. Although they were young women at the time, 17 and 20, and we are very close, I knew this would be a real shock in their lives. When I left the outpatient area after the first surgery and had a pretty good idea that it was cancer, I still decided not to tell them until I was sure.

My youngest daughter, Lacey, was living at home so even though she and her sister knew that I was going to have surgery, I tried to "play it down" so she wouldn't worry. Keep in mind that I really didn't know that it WAS serious, and I felt there was no reason to worry anyone yet. My oldest daughter was attending a conference in Nashville until Sunday so I knew I wouldn't have to tell her anything until she got back to her apartment. All I really had to deal with at this time was my youngest daughter, and my very closest friends.

When I came home from the hospital, I told Lacey that the surgery went well, and that we wouldn't really know anything for sure until Thursday when I went to the doctor. I still didn't feel it was necessary to worry her until I had some additional answers regarding prognosis, procedure, etc. The surgery was on Monday. By Wednesday, the day before my appointment with Dr. B, I mentioned that the doctor thought it might be cancer, but didn't know for sure. I believe this brief statement helped plant a little seed so that when I came home the next day with a long diagnosis and prognosis, it wouldn't overwhelm her – at least that was my thought.

Mary, my pinky swear friend stopped by the hospital before the surgery so I knew I had to talk with her and tell her what the doctor said. That was one of the first difficult calls. She handled it very well and knew that my attitude needed to remain up and strong so the warm feeling of support was evident (even though I know now that she was faking it!).

As it turned out, Lacey handled it as well as any seventeen year old could have given the same situation. I was already doing the best to prepare myself, and had already called in some of the Humor Team members since Dr. B told me what he thought. By the time I had talked to Lacey, I had already made the decision that I couldn't change the diagnosis, but I had a choice on how I wanted to respond, and that response was going to be as positive as I could possibly be. I tried my very best to be positive when I told Lacey all the information Dr. B had delivered. In reality, things could have been a lot worse. If I had cancelled the mammogram appointment...If we hadn't caught the cancer early... If I didn't have confidence in my doctor, etc. I think the positive way I told her had a bearing on the way she accepted the information. She cried a little, but we talked more than anything. I knew there would be tears for her later, as there were for me, and I made sure she understood that it was okay if she felt she needed to cry, or talk, or whatever. Overall, it went as well as could be expected.

One of the most difficult people to tell was going to be my mother. We are very close; in fact she constantly tells me I am her favorite daughter. Okay, okay, I am her only daughter! She was in the middle of a 3½ week trip across the United States! I did not tell her that I was going in for the biopsy before she left because I did not want her to cancel the trip and worry needlessly. Now that I was fairly sure it was cancer, this was another matter. However, I had a plan!

It turned out that the last week of her trip was going to be spent with my aunt and uncle in their Phoenix home. My aunt had gone through breast cancer just two years ago, and, most importantly, had an excellent attitude. How she viewed her journey with cancer was very important to me when I thought of people I could talk to at this crucial time. I didn't want to know about her surgery or treatment, as I was already subconsciously building my shield that I talked about earlier, but what I wanted and needed from her was her positive attitude. We both shared the idea that we couldn't change it, but we could choose how we responded to the diagnosis.

My mother was scheduled to arrive on Thursday, the same day I met with Dr. B for the diagnosis and prognosis. The plan was to call my aunt and uncle on Saturday morning and talk with my mom. There was no reason to call on her first night there and put a damper on this part of her vacation – she couldn't change it either. Also, this way my aunt and uncle, who are both very positive people, would be there for her. Even if I had told her when she was in her own home, we live nearly 400 miles away from each other and she would have still been alone when I called. This way she would not only have supportive family close, but people who knew first hand about the experience with breast cancer.

Well, you know about the best-laid plans. As it turned out, my mother called me while I was at Dr. B's and left a message on my voice mail at work. I was hoping I still wouldn't need to talk to her until Saturday, but she called me back later Thursday evening. I couldn't put it off any longer.

After an extended conversation about her trip and all of the beautiful things she was seeing, I told her I had something to tell her, and I just went on with the story! Don't get me wrong about my mother. She is a recently retired nurse, and a very sharp woman. She is not weak or wimpy, but when it comes to your own daughter, and, remember, I AM her favorite, something like this out of the clear blue is totally unexpected and a shock. Besides, even my mother knows that I am statistically too young to have breast cancer. Geez, I always did hate statistics in school!!!

I told her I had something to tell her. The statement was simply, "Mom, I have been diagnosed with breast cancer, and I need you on my Humor Team." She took everything well, but I could tell she was crying. I just went on and on with the story, including adding the characters names, you know, Inny and how I would now have to change it to "Stitchette" or something, and about Dr. B saying he would put a gold tassle in if I brought it to the surgery, and everything else positive I could think of at the time. She asked a lot of questions and I gave her all the answers I had at the time. When we ended the conversation she seemed okay with everything and we said the usual "I love you'" and hung up. Another one down.

I called her back on Saturday to make sure everything was still okay. One of the first things she said to me was, "Are you sure you're telling me everything? You're not hiding anything?" I must have been convincing (and I wasn't hiding anything!) and the conversation ended on a positive note.

When you're faced with a situation like this, keep in mind that this is very personal and YOU choose who you tell. Beware though of the people you tell who think they are saving you from having to go through this again, and they tell the whole world for you! I knew this would eventually happen in my workplace, but for the time being I chose the co-workers I wanted to know. I told them over a series of days, and I only told the parts I wanted to share.

As I mentioned, my oldest daughter, Tiffany, was away at a conference and I didn't get a chance to tell her until Monday, a week after the biopsy. I started by asking her how her trip went, and that took a very long time. From a bomb threat, to a robbery, to an anthrax scare and a tornado (I think I will let her write her own story!!), it took a while to get caught up on her life. Then, I basically went through the same procedure as I did with Mom, and got the same response! Tiffany was quietly crying and I was talking and talking!! I was trying to let her know that I had decided to tackle this situation with all the "comedic mustard" I could find!! I was not going to let this get me down – I was going to fight and conquer!!! I think I was realizing that the more I said it, the more I became convinced that it was reality – and it was!! Another step on the path to my personal recovery! I believe my reassuring attitude helped her to understand what I was saying and how I was coping, even if she didn't really believe me. I also knew there would be later tears for her as it started to sink in and I repeated the open door policy on talking, tears, and laughter!

    I continued to tell close friends, and I made a very interesting discovery. It seemed as though the people I told in person responded better overall than the people I told over the phone. As a student and teacher of communication, I believe it was because they could see from the look in my eyes and my body gestures that I was very serious about my chosen lighter approach to this situation. My advice to anyone facing such a situation is that it is better if at all possible to tell people in person, most importantly if you have also chosen the positive approach, as it helps them by drawing from and forging with your strength. Over the phone, there isn't the possibility of seeing, hugging, and holding to gain that strength they may need.

    I found I spent a lot of time reassuring others that I was really going to be okay. This seemed so weird and bizarre as I was the one who had the cancer, but I had the advantage in making my choice to be positive, while others weren't sure if that was okay yet or not.

Lesson Ten *– Be informed! There is a ton of information out there about breast cancer. See what your doctor recommends. Take the books home and read, read, and re-read the information. For me personally, I found the publications from the American Cancer Society and the National Institute of Health very helpful. The information was in simple terms that I could understand. Unless you have personally studied medicine, there are a lot of new terms that you will hear and you HAVE to understand them to make the best decisions. Although I offer lists of questions to ask at various stages, these books will help you develop your own list of important questions to ask.*

Chapter Ten
The "Big" Surgery

"What lies before us and what lies behind us are tiny matters compared to what lies within us."
— Ralph Waldo Emerson

    The day of my "big" surgery was filled with all kinds of excitement. As I mentioned before, I had already stopped in to talk to the anesthesiologist and nursing staff so I knew what to expect.

    My mother had come in from Ohio to be with me during the surgery and for a few days afterwards to make sure everything went well. She is a registered nurse and a very strong person. One of my biggest concerns when she said she would be taking care of me, was that she would take "too" good of care of me. This may sound strange but it goes back to control issue that we have previously discussed. There was so much happening around me since I was diagnosed and so much to think about that I felt like my life was spinning out of control. I was holding on to anything at all that I felt was within my control. My poor mother, when she first arrived, I told her I was really glad that she was here, but I needed to talk with the doctor and make my own decisions. What I was really afraid of is that she would ask all kinds of technical questions and I wouldn't understand what she and Dr. B were talking about. In other words, I wouldn't be in control. However, being a mother myself, I fully understood the need for a mother to take care of her daughter, and in this case, her <u>favorite</u> daughter (I DID mention that I am my mother's only daughter, right?!).

I needed to document everything that was happening, both in words and pictures. Since my physical appearance would be forever changed after the surgery, I wanted pictures of the before and after. This may sound a bit morbid, but you have to do what is right for <u>you</u>. For me, this permanent change was very important and for some reason the photographs became an important part of the journey.

You Light Up My Life

The day started with a few minutes in the surgical area, and then I was whisked off to the Nuclear Medicine department. I remember the Nuclear Medicine department was decorated with soft pink colors and it just "felt" warm and caring. I found out that the room matched the personalities of the people working in this department.

All that was happening was new (thankfully) and actually interesting. Again, I just wish it was happening to someone else.

I was introduced to the entire staff and we started to joke around about the stove pipe hat I had on my head with "Tammy's Team" and the clown noses I had brought along. I didn't go anywhere in the hospital without my supply of noses!

As it turned out, the Radiologist was a huge Three Stooges fan, so we had a good laugh about the noses and shared our favorite episodes of the Three Stooges. Everyone was so very kind, but there is one young woman who will be forever etched in my mind.

"I'll Be Right Here to Hold Your Hand"

The reason I was in this department was to have a procedure whereby I was injected with radioactive isotopes for a procedure called a Sentinel Node Biopsy. The idea of his procedure is that the lymphatic vessels carry the dye to the "sentinel" (or main) lymph node. During the surgery, the doctor can then see the dye and detect the radioactivity with a Geiger counter (cool – just like a hidden treasure!), then they can cut this part out and have it examined right there during the operation. The advantage of this procedure is that they no longer have to arbitrarily take all of the lymph nodes out, which can be a very painful, and in some cases unnecessary surgery. The piece that is removed can be examined and a determination can be made to recommend removing other lymph nodes or not, depending on the test results.

The radioactive isotopes are injected directly into the affected site. Since my cancer was right at the nipple, this is where the shots needed to be administered. This young woman, Lori, was standing right beside my head. She told me that depending on where the shots were administered would determine the amount of associated pain. When she found out it was directly in the nipple, she took my hand and said, "This is really going to hurt, and I am going to stand right here and hold your hand. You just squeeze as hard as you like, I am going to be right here." You hear so much about people in the medical field and that the "personal touching" is sometimes not acceptable behavior. I can tell you from this situation that I am so glad that Lori believed in the personal touch, because as a patient, it made a huge difference in my experience on the bed that day. Lori also mentioned that she had just had surgery three weeks before, and knew what a difference the attitudes of the people taking care of her made in both her procedure and the recovery.

The first four shots were a little painful, but the fifth shot seemed to strike a nerve, or something. Whatever it was, it was extremely painful and I started to tear up.

More than Just Getting Through

I was still in quite a bit of pain from the injections when they had to take x-rays of the isotopes as they settled into the affected area. This part of the procedure involved a square frame, approximately 12 inches by 12 inches to come down, very, very close to my body and take the x-ray. I am extremely claustrophobic, but I can usually get through procedures like this if I keep my eyes closed. I am sure it was a combination of being scared, uncertain, and hurting, but I made the mistake of opening my eyes for a split second. Keep in mind that this square was the only part covering me and all around me was open. It didn't seem to matter; I panicked and started yelling for them to "let me out". They instantly lifted the machine and the doctor immediately was at my side with his hand on my shoulder telling me it was okay, not to worry, he was one of the most claustrophobic people in the hospital and understood completely. We would just try it again in a few minutes when I was ready. This may not seem like much to you as you are reading this, but the compassion shown by this doctor and staff was exceptional. The next time through they gave me a washcloth to put over my eyes and we got through the procedure without incident.

At the end of the procedure, everyone came out of the little room where they "hide" during an x-ray wearing their clown noses and we had a great laugh! Lori asked me if I had any extra noses, as they occasionally get children in the department, and she felt the noses would make for a lighter time for children undergoing a very scary procedure. I made sure she had a couple of extra noses, but reminded her that you just have to be a child at heart to appreciate the levity that a clown nose can bring to a room – it certainly worked for me – and THEM.

I told them that I was planning to write a book about the journey. They asked if there were any questions, showed me the films, and explained in great detail what they were doing and what was happening in my body. Their attitudes and compassion made a great deal of difference with this procedure. I mention many people throughout this book who made a difference along my path, but I cannot say enough how important that was to me as a patient. Clearly, this is their "job", but so many of the people I met along the way went way beyond their "job" and went that extra step to show personal commitment and compassion for the patient. When this happens to you, whether it is healthcare or otherwise, please make sure you remember to say "thank you". It can certainly make a difference in their lives, too.

Back to the Waiting Room

The above procedure can take quite a long time, depending on how the body responds to the dye, therefore, they generally allow a couple of hours for the procedure in the preparation time before surgery. As it turned out, my body responded very well to the procedure and I was done in less than an hour. Since that was the case, I returned to the surgery area to wait for the actual procedure to begin.

Sitting in the waiting room, we all had on the stovepipe hats that were made to wear to Dr. Schrock's presentation with the "Tammy's Team" bands. There were kazoos playing softly every now and then, and the red noses graced our faces as people walked by in the hallway. We were certainly a wild bunch of people, but to the others sharing the waiting room, it seemed to make a difference, and it certainly was helping the time pass for me.

During the time that I was waiting, I decided that I should grace my breasts with a little artwork for Dr. B. By the time he saw me for the first time, I had already taken a marker and drew multi-colored hearts and little notes, like "Hi! Dr. B" and "This one" with arrows on the left breast.

My Humor Team had decided that I needed a good send-off to surgery, so they had arranged a time to give me a kazoo send-off. When the nurse called me back into the room for the preparations, my Humor Team delightfully broke out in song with MY MANTRA on the kazoo!!! It had to be the best send-off into surgery a person has ever had!

My Right Mind?

The anesthesiologist, Dr. M, was absolutely fantastic. I had met with him the week before the surgery, and we had discussed all the options. I was very comfortable with the procedure by this time and was ready to get on with it. The procedure was relatively painless and the medication started to take effect very quickly.

I had brought along a stovepipe hat for Dr. B and for some reason I was afraid that my mother or CJ, would forget to give it to him. CJ tells me that I asked him "several" times about the hat and to make sure that Dr. B saw it before we went in. To this day I don't understand what I was thinking, but I am always ribbed about being so adamant about "the hat". The only plea I have is temporary drug-induced insanity.

The one regret I have is that I wish I would have worn my big red clown shoes into surgery. The image of those big shoes under the sheets still makes me chuckle! However, I pray there won't be a "next time", so I will just have to live vicariously through the image!

A Prayerful Moment

By the time Dr. B came into the room, I was feeling very *good*, if you know what I mean, but I still had enough faculties to know the deep value of what was about to happen. My mother was beside my bed when Dr. B came in and asked if I had any questions. By this time all of my questions had been sufficiently answered and there was only one thing left to do. I took Dr. B's hand and asked him if he would pray with me. There wasn't a second of hesitation and I briefly said a quick prayer and we were on our way.

The deep value of this very quick exchange was that Dr. B was praying with ME because I was the patient and I felt that I needed it to get through the surgery. It didn't matter what religion Dr. B was, he was most concerned about ME, the patient in this exchange. This single moment was so important in my overall view and respect of Dr. B and I will never forget this generosity. The prayer was for God to bless Dr. B as he performed the surgery, and I certainly felt blessed.

The Laughing Club

Although Dr. M administered the initial spinal block, the anesthesiologist who wheeled me back to the operating room was Dr. V. On my bed I had a full supply of noses for the operating staff and the "Tammy's Team" hat for Dr. B. I was handing out noses to everyone we met and Dr. V was laughing about the nose exchange. As he was wheeling me down the hall, he told me that he was originally from India and his parents were still living there. A few times a week they went to the beach to join a very large group of people in a "Laughing Club". The whole idea was to get together and laugh for a short while then go back home feeling rejuvenated and refreshed. Both of his parents were in their late 80's and very healthy, and they felt their involvement with the "Laughing Club" was in part what kept them strong and healthy.

Calling All Clowns

While I was in the operating room, a few of my clown friends stopped by, in costume, to sit with my family. Well, actually, there wasn't any sitting going on. From what I heard afterwards and the pictures I saw, they were having a grand time while I was in surgery. It is amazing how a couple of clowns in the waiting room can make a difference in how the time passes when you are concerned about a loved one. While I do some hospital clowning, there are clowns in our clown group who clown at the hospital on a weekly basis. To all of them, I say "thank you" from my family for helping others to see this part of the lighter side of recovery!

Hmmm, A Warm Blanket!

It is funny how we can remember the smallest gesture when we are dealing with some traumatic event in our lives. I have already expressed some of the caring gestures from people throughout this journey, but Dr. V provided another one as I was coming out of the anesthetic. I remember I was so TERRIBLY cold and I distinctly remember Dr. V (the anesthesiologist) wrapping a warm blanket around my shoulders and face to warm me. His soft voice and the warmth of the blankets certainly eased any concerns I had at the immediate time. A small gesture that meant so very much!

A Party at MY Bedside

I obviously don't remember much about the surgery, except for coming out of the anesthetic and hearing Dr. B's voice. It was a welcome voice, and I knew I had safely made it through the surgery.

I was taken to the recovery room and as I slowly came out of the anesthetic, I realized there were three or four people standing around my bed – LAUGHING!!! I certainly didn't want to miss anything, and this laughter seemed to involve ME!!! As it turned out, Dr. B felt that he couldn't give me an actual "smile" incision, so he drew a smiley face where the incision was AND a very large Mickey Mouse head on the upper side of the bandage!!! He used a deep purple marker and it was very easy for everyone to see!! What a riot!

I was still a little groggy and would close my eyes from time to time. I heard Dr. B's voice as he came into the recovery room and as I opened my eyes, he was looking down at me WITH A CLOWN NOSE ON!! If that isn't a sight to behold as you are coming out from anesthetic, I don't know what is! I thought maybe I had died and gone to heaven and there ARE clowns in heaven!!

He told me the surgery went very well and the lymph nodes looked cancer-free. I thanked God for that piece of good news!

A Talk with the Family

The entire surgery took a little over 2½ hours. After the surgery my family was asked to meet Dr. B in a little room outside of the waiting room. Thankfully, Dr. B's nurse had already told me this was going to happen. Where most doctors talk to the family in the waiting room, Dr. B likes to have a little more privacy for the family and friends waiting. Had he not told us this, I am sure my family would have panicked that something has gone terribly wrong.

Obviously, I was not part of this conversation, but from what I am told, Dr. B was very positive about the surgery and told my family that the surgery went well, and it looked like there was no cancer in the lymph nodes. As it turned out later, the more advanced test showed something else, but I will talk about that in an upcoming chapter.

Just Call Me Mama Smurf

After I was coherent in the recovery room, they moved me to another room to monitor my vital signs and determine whether or not I could go home that night or if I needed to stay until morning. According to my mother, I had already decided "I was out of there" and was very adamant that I was going home, but it took the staff a little while to reach the same conclusion.

While I was waiting, everyone kept laughing at me because my skin tone was actually blue!!! No, I don't mean a little blue, but REALLY blue!! I looked like Mama Smurf! (If you are not sure what a "Smurf" is, they were little cartoon characters that were a vibrant blue color.) As it turned out, the dyes that they used in the Nuclear Medicine department are blue so that the doctor can see them easier during surgery. This certainly works out of your system, but it takes a little while. In the meantime, I was actually blue! I kind of had a Ty-D-Bol effect for a while, if you know what I mean. You know, you just can't make this stuff up!!!

Recovery, Shop-a-holic Style

I had a very restful night once I got home, sore, but restful. My mother was staying with me for a few days so the next day we did what we both do best and that is SHOPPING!!!

Dr. B didn't really put any restrictions on me except to avoid heavy lifting for a while, and I figured it wouldn't take much to lift a credit card out of my wallet! Mom and I headed out to the mall, me fully bandaged and toting ice packs! Remember, I told you she was a nurse, and, in fact, had been a recovery room nurse for quite a while in her career. What better person to help me with the initial recovery than a trained professional? Actually, if the truth be known, she wasn't dragging me out the door; I think I was taking the lead!

In all honesty, I think I wanted to shop so that I would feel "alive"! I wanted to be out with people and walk around like a "normal" person. Shopping has always had therapeutic effects for both me and my Mom, and the fact that we were doing it together at this time really meant more than just going to the mall.

Recouping

I was only off work a couple of days from the surgery. My Mom had gone back to Ohio, and CJ and Lacey were helping to take care of the little things I needed at home. It was important for me to get back to doing the normal routine as soon as possible.

I had to be careful not to bump my chest or left arm. Well, actually the greater danger for me was to watch that the cats or dog didn't jump on my chest on the way to the open window at night! That only happened once and I can assure you I was thoroughly protected from that point on!

For the most part, people didn't even know that anything had happened. Two days after the surgery I was back teaching a class, and, even though CJ went along in case I needed a back up, I was actually able to conduct the class without a problem. This particular class was a group of women from the banking industry. When I came to class, there were all kinds of questions about the procedure, how I discovered it, and what I had learned about breast cancer. It was obvious that most of these women had never discussed this issue with anyone who had personally experienced breast cancer. As it turned out, it was really great for me to talk about the experience and helpful for them to see someone who was dealing with this in a positive upbeat manner. In fact, several months after this class I received a lovely note from one of my students thanking me for the frank discussion that evening and saying that it had made such an impact on her life that she scheduled a mammogram the next day and her mother did too! Even if we help just one person, we are making a difference.

NO WAY!!!

Within a week after my mother left, she found herself in HER doctor's office for a lump in her breast!! When she told me I could not believe the irony. Thank God that it turned out to be nothing to worry about, but I will tell you, I was already lining people up for HER Humor Team!!

Another Recovery Ditty

To get the full effect of this section, it is best to be familiar with the Mounds (oh, so appropriate) and Almond Joy candy bar commercials. The words to the commercial are:

> Sometimes you feel like a nut,
> Sometimes you don't.
> Almond Joy has nuts
> Mounds don't
> Because....
> Sometimes you feel like a nut,
> Sometimes you don't!

For some strange reason, after the surgery was over, and all bandages were removed, one day this commercial came into my mind, but the words weren't exactly the same (I know, you're surprised!). Instead, my recovery ditty went something like this:

> Sometimes you feel like a "nip",
> Sometimes you don't.
> One breast has a "nip"

One breast don't
Because....
Sometimes you feel like a "nip",
Sometimes you don't!

There were also some simple hand gestures to accompany the song, but they are not required to be a little crazy! Admittedly, it was not a common song, but it did and still does bring a smile to my face every time I hear the original commercial!

Bandages Off!

When all of the bandages finally came off, I was really surprised at the new appearance of my breast. I wasn't sure what to expect, but it turned out that the incision was about 2½ inches long and was almost horizontally straight across my breast. As it healed through time, the scar became less and less noticeable, and if you were to see the breast out of context, it may be very difficult to even see the scar.

Lesson Eleven *– Remain positive in every way that you can, no matter how small. The benefits of positive thoughts are scientifically proven to far outweigh negative thoughts on the road to recovery. Remember, you have a CHOICE on how you respond. No one says it will be easy but, once you set the attitude to succeed, stay with it and remind yourself constantly that the benefits of this positive attitude extend far beyond the immediate, and are a key to your successful recovery. Yes, I know I already said this, but when something must be remembered, it is important to see it at least three times before it truly becomes a mental habit.*

Chapter Eleven
Just Call Me Dolly

"To be a star, you must shine your own light, follow your own path, and don't worry about the darkness, for that is when the stars shine brightest." — Unknown Author

It is amazing the different types of stories the wig buying and wearing experience brought about. As I mentioned before, Dolly Parton is one of my favorite performers. If someone were to ask me who I would really like to meet in life, at least in the entertainment business, it would clearly be Dolly and Carol Burnett. There is truly a gift in the ability to make others laugh, and I think both of these women have that special gift.

Although I have never seen Dolly perform in person, I have listened to her personal autobiography and her songs for many years. There is just something about her that speaks to me. I think part of it is her personal story. When she talks about her childhood, I think of my own mother's childhood and I believe there is some sort of invisible connection.

This might be because my mother's side of the family is from the hills of West Virginia and Kentucky, or maybe because I have always loved blond hair, who knows why, but I have always been fascinated by Dolly Parton. I have spent many hours listening to her read her autobiography on tape, and have enjoyed the way she paints a picture with her words that so easily transports the listener to the Smoky Mountains of her youth. And even though I am not a true country music fan, I have always enjoyed listening to her sing one of the more than 400 songs that she has written and published. Again, whatever the reason, I have always liked Dolly and she is on my goal list to meet some day. (In case you're reading this Dolly, just give me a call anytime and I will clear my calendar!!).

Now, having said that, there is a reason I bring Dolly into this story. When the idea of facing chemo was very real, and I was thinking about a shunt vs. IV, and how I might lose my hair, and what type of shining agent I could use, I thought about getting a wig. I felt that I was strong enough to face some parts of the day without any hair, but I knew there would be times at work or going out that I would feel more comfortable with a wig.

I started my search as I normally would – in a strange place. Actually, my search started me! I wasn't even thinking about getting a wig when I came across a beautiful little wig in a thrift store, one of my very favorite shopping spots. It was a different color than my own hair, but I felt it was in excellent condition, and for $2.00 I couldn't go wrong. Besides, a nice change in hair color every now and then should be fun. Let's face it, as Hugz the Clown, the flaming red hair that I wear as part of my costume always gives me a lift. There seems to be therapy in being someone else for a little while.

You may know that one of the terrible side effects of chemotherapy is total hair loss for many people. This can be doubly traumatic for women, and a lot of women go in search of a wig that matches their natural (or in my case – bottled) hair color before beginning the chemotherapy. As it turns out, I was shopping in an area mall shortly after Halloween and came across a costume shop going out of business. It was the type of shop that is only open for the Halloween season. While a suitable wig may not be found in most costume shops, the shop I stumbled across was not the usual costume shop! This shop had wigs of all shapes and colors, and quite frankly, some were downright SEXY!!! Yes! Right up my alley!!!

These were not your ordinary, everyday wigs, but what I would call "glamour" wigs. There were long brunettes, red heads, silver manes, Marilyn Monroes, and Sophia Lorens. I saw wigs of all shapes and colors, but the one that caught my eye was way up near the ceiling, on a foam head – and it was pure DOLLY!!!! I just had to try this wig on. I gently lifted the beautiful blond locks off of the foam head and headed for the mirror. WOW!!!! This was really a full, full wig!! In fact, I think the first time I looked in the mirror, I didn't even recognize myself! It was beautiful. CJ was with me, and I could tell by the look on his face that he felt it should stay "way up by the ceiling" in the shop, but I didn't let his look dissuade me, and I knew it was a keeper. I knew if I didn't buy it on the spot, I would always regret it. The price was right, and the spirit was right, so this beautiful wig came home with me that day! You already know my theory – I couldn't change what was going to happen, but I was in control of how I responded, and Dolly and I were responding – big time (actually big curly wig, big time)!

In her autobiography, Dolly talks about why she loves to wear wigs. She says she really enjoys being able to have her hair done, and she doesn't have to be there – what a neat idea!

When I took the wig to the counter the young sales girl commented on how beautiful it was and I told her I was getting ready to receive chemotherapy and, if it was going to happen, I was going to make the best of the situation. I think she thought I was kidding at first, but when she realized that I was serious, we both laughed about taking on the town, Dolly-style.

I work in a company with about 1,000 employees, and, as a clown, I have been known to dress a little strange from time to time and do some things that the traditional person may not partake in on a regular basis. I say this because my Dolly wig created quite a stir that actually taught me a valuable lesson. I brought my wig to work to try on and see if I liked the look and feel in the office setting. I was talking with a few co-workers in the hall, when another of my co-workers (not a close one) passed me and said, "Freak". I could not believe he had made that comment, but sure enough he did. I asked him why he called me such a name and he said, "You just look like one. What are you doing, going to a costume party?" I was a little upset at his callous remark and simply responded, "No, as a matter of fact, I am getting ready to start chemo for cancer and wanted to see what the wig looked like before I actually needed it." And I added, "You might want to have all the facts before you call someone a name." The women who were standing around me when he walked by gave me a "high-five" and we continued our conversation. The lesson I learned that day was actually a reminder to myself to gather all of the facts before I open my mouth to insert my foot! Shoe leather just does not have a very good taste. This person did apologize to me later, but I hope he learned this valuable lesson, too. Especially since he has children at home who can be very impressionable.

Although I had my Dolly wig, I also thought it would be nice to have a smaller, casual wig. The town I live in is not very big, but I found a shop in a neighboring town and decided to visit to see what was available. I thought this would be a simple trip to the boutique, but it was a horrific experience. To this day I wish I would have reported the woman who *waited* on me (and I use this term loosely). Although she said she was a survivor, she was a terrible person to have in a position that took care of women with a wig need, especially because of an associated illness. She was nasty and snappy and I walked out of the store so angry that it still makes my blood heat up when I think about her. I try to give people the benefit of the doubt that they are having a bad day but this woman must have been having a bad decade! In fact, as I was stewing outside of the doorway, another woman walked by and said, "She is always like that". The moral of this part of my story is another valuable lesson. There are a lot of places out there, no matter where you live – DO NOT allow people to treat you poorly – you have a choice here, too! I did find another, smaller wig to wear for "less than Dolly" situations at another shop that looked very nice and natural. I have told anyone who would listen not to deal with this woman and this wig boutique.

Thanks, Dolly, for helping to teach me these valuable lessons!

Lesson Twelve - WRITE down the questions that you want to ask, and be ready to record the answers! Keep a notebook with you at all times, especially beside the bed for when the questions come to mind. Jot them down immediately and then, if it is something you can look up in the reading material, fine. If not, you have it to record on the main list you take with you when you talk to your doctor.

Chapter Twelve
Office Visits

"The most wasted of all days is one without laughter."

- e.e.cummings

I have already given you my impression of the first time I met Dr. B, but I haven't really told you what others had to say about him. Everyone I had talked to up to that point had only good comments to say about him. Many people said his bedside manner was a little uptight, but he was a well-respected and excellent doctor. The idea that he was considered by some to be a little stiff made the next experience all the sweeter. At the end of the second visit to Dr. B's office, he ended the visit by saying, "By the way, I wore my clown nose into a patient's room the other day." I think I hear harp music playing some place – the subtle differences we make in the lives of others!

All of the office visits to Dr. B's office became great adventures after the first visit. Since I started with clown noses and a Humor Team, it was difficult to just walk in like a "normal" patient. This whole concept became quite a fun challenge, and a lot of hard work!

One day as I was sitting at home recovering after the partial mastectomy, I was playing with some "Sculpty" modeling clay. This is a very pliable clay that comes in many colors and has many uses, but I am not sure it has ever been used for the purpose I was about to use it for!!! During the conversations with Dr. B about reconstruction, we talked about the option of a prosthesis, however since I was losing the front part of the breast, I wouldn't really need an entire prosthetic piece. It may sound silly, but I thought there might be occasions that I would like to have just a nipple. Quite frankly, I can't think of any right off hand, but you never know. I certainly couldn't justify having something like this specially made, but if I could make one….

I got a pack of "Sculpty" at the local craft store and mixed a couple of colors together until it was close to my skin tone. I then sat and molded the clay into what I thought resembled a two-piece nipple. It took a few tries, but by the third try, I had something that actually looked like a real nipple. I kept the first two attempts, so I actually had a collection of three nipples. Now, what to do with them?

On my next visit to Dr. B's office, I took some liquid adhesive that I use to apply my rubber clown nose, and applied ALL THREE nipples to my breast area! When Dr. B came in the room I said, "Dr. B, I know you are the expert and I don't claim to be, but is this normal?" Oh, I wish I had a camera!!!! The look on his face was priceless!! He tried desperately to keep a straight face and turned and mumbled something about, "If I didn't know you so well, I would REALLY be worried." I still laugh and laugh when I think of that visit!!

On another visit he walked through the door and I was wearing a REALLY UGLY big rubber Halloween mask. I had tried it on the crew in Radiology and it worked very well, so I thought I would give it a go with Dr. B. He didn't disappoint me!! He gasped and said he knew to expect something, but this even had him surprised!

There were visits with wigs, and hats, and feather boas, and wild glasses, just to name a few. It got to the point that I was glad when the visits weren't so often – I was getting exhausted thinking of new ideas.

Not only was the plan to help Dr. B, his nurse, and staff with a little levity, but it was also therapeutic for me to continually remind myself that I was alive and was (and AM) celebrating this life!!!

What?? It's Missing???

The time rolled around for the first follow-up mammogram after being diagnosed. I can certainly say that I was a little anxious about the results, but I knew that no matter what happened, I could face it – I had already been there before and had a much better idea of what to expect.

I checked in with the receptionist, went to the dressing room, changed my clothes and sat in the waiting room. A couple of time I felt especially anxious, but started to hum my mantra and that calmed me considerably.

When the young woman came to get me from the waiting room she was very sweet and we talked and joked on the way back to the mammogram machine. If you have had a mammogram, then you will know what I am referring to when I talk about the little metal "sticky BB's". If not, let me quickly explain that when you get a mammogram, a small round circle with a metal ball in the middle, similar to a BB is placed on the nipple so that it shows on the mammogram film. This allows the therapist to see exactly where the nipple is located in comparison to the rest of the breast.

This lovely young woman must not have looked at my file before taking me into the room. As I slipped off my gown, she said, "Now, this will only take a minute. Let me place these on you and we will get started." She came at me with two stickers ready to be appropriately placed. As I turned toward her she looked at my breast and said, "Oh, you only have one nipple." I looked at her, straight in the eyes and replied with a frantic face, "What??!! I am missing a nipple??!!" The look on her face was priceless! She truly did not know what to say, but when she responded, "Umm, you did know that, right?", it was just too much and I burst out laughing. She joined me in laughter and we had a good time laughing at the silliness.

Still looking for opportunities to laugh…..

Lesson Thirteen – Look for the smallest blessings in each day. No matter what we are facing, there is always something to be thankful for. It could be a person, or a hug or kind word, or a card received, or the sun shining through the window. Each day offers a multitude of blessing that we can each count, but sometimes we get so caught up in what we are dealing with, that we forget the little things that can make a big difference. Look for them – they are everywhere.

Chapter Thirteen
Signs from God

"Your talent is God's gift to you. What you do with it is your gift back to God."
— Leo Buscaglia

I am a person who strongly believes in signs from God. Perhaps you have similar beliefs that may or may not involve God, but there were clearly a few signs along my path that were so obvious that even I understood their value. Some people believe in coincidence. I do not. I believe everything happens for a reason, some reasons we understand quickly. Others we understand over time. Yet others, we may never understand why they happened.

One of the "biggest" signs, in a couple of ways, happened along a major interstate as I was traveling to do a workshop. During the early part of my journey, I had a lot of decisions to make. Your doctors, family, and friends can offer you choices, but you ultimately have to make a lot of the decisions by yourself. This decision making can be one of the most traumatic experiences of this whole journey.

I was driving on the highway, praying to God that I was making the right decisions. I often believe that I am so dense that I can easily miss the signs along the way. This particular day, I was praying, "Please God, send me a sign that you are with me and that I am making the right decisions. And, God, you know I don't always understand what You want me to know, so please make it something big so there is no question. Please send me a big sign so there is no doubt." As I rounded the curve, there was the largest "sign" I have ever seen. It was a new highway sign they were trying out for the local baseball field game traffic. It was a huge sign that was ultimately to be attached to a large pole – placing it many feet above the highway, but that day it wasn't about a ball game, it was a sign for me from God. I had specifically asked for a big sign, one that I understood, and resting on the side of the road this sign (probably 6 feet by 15 feet) was huge. I laughed and cried at the sight of "my" big sign, and, to this day, each time I pass one of these signs, the tears come to my eyes in thankfulness for this message from God.

When I was first diagnosed with cancer, I was in the process of leaving my full-time job and working part-time for the local Small Business Development Center. I had been doing my speaking business along with my clowning and full-time job, but I decided I wanted to try the speaking business full-time. I was in touch with the local Small Business Development Center with my business and it turned out they had a position that would meet both our needs. Since the job was part-time, there wasn't any insurance provided with the position. Before I made this change, knowing I wouldn't have insurance coverage for a while, I decided to have a thorough physical. It was during this physical that my cancer was discovered. I have always been thankful that it was discovered when it was, or the outcome may have been different.

The day after I told the women at the Small Business Development Center that I was facing cancer and wouldn't be coming to work with them, I received the following message from one of them regarding the Dr. Schrock seminar I mentioned earlier:

> "Ok - you're the one always saying you don't believe in coincidences - this came in today on a listserv (an e-mail group) I didn't even know I belonged to. So I'm passing it along. I doubt there's anyone who is more positive than you though. I don't know why things like this happen. But they do. At this point your health is of course paramount to anything else. Please keep in touch. We care, Linda"

I especially enjoyed the part about "not believing in coincidences".

From the diagnosis through the three surgeries and the treatments, I was nightly reading a book that seemed to be "speaking" to me. The book was Norman Vincent Peale's, "In God We Trust". Each chapter that I read seemed to deal with <u>exactly</u> what I was feeling – worry, concern, thankfulness, even dying. One night the verse was, "This is the Day the Lord hath made, rejoice and be glad in it. " I went to bed with that in my head and heart and that was the first thought I had when I awoke the next morning. There were so many emotions flowing. Later that day I spoke to my friend Julia who is a very spiritual person. She had just found out the day before about my diagnosis. She was very upset and prayed to God to give her the right words to say. She said the words did not come that day, but this particular morning when she woke she prayed again and God sent her a direct message for me. He told her to remind me that (you guessed it!), "This is the day the Lord hath made, rejoice and be glad in it"!!! . (Since the time I started the book, Julia has also become a breast cancer survivor!)

After the surgeries and shortly before I started the radiation, I was walking into work reflecting on the events of the past few months. When I got into my office, I received this message from a good friend:

Tammy:

Hello there! For some reason you're popping into my mind quite often lately. Please know that I've been thinking and praying for you. I feel led to encourage you but not quite sure what to say. I do want to remind you that you're very special and I admire you. You're an awesome person! I always feel uplifted after talking to you or being around you. You've been an inspiration to me and I'm very thankful that we're friends. I pray that you're doing well. Hang in there...things will get better.

Love ya,
Faithann

It was clearly messages like these that I held close and cherished. It seemed as though any time I was feeling down, God would put someone on my path or send me a message to remind me that I was never alone and that I needed to keep going.

Across the Airwaves

After I met with Dr. D in Radiology, I had to decide whether or not to have the lymph nodes radiated. I had done my research and knew there was a risk of a condition called lymphedema, which can be a very painful swelling of the lymph nodes. I had chosen not to have all of the lymph nodes removed after the surgery, but there was the question of including them in the radiation. It was another major decision and I was in a state of exhaustion. As I mentioned, the medication-induced hot flashes were preventing me from sleeping and I was thoroughly spent. I had to make the decision within the next half hour and as much as I had been praying about it, still didn't know what to do. I felt completely frustrated and scared. I was praying as I got in the car to drive to the appointment. I was already on my way to the appointment so it didn't matter what research I had done or anything else, I had to make a decision and there was no place left, at least in my mind, that God could give me direction. I got in the car and the local Christian radio station, WTLR, was on the radio. The topic was women and faith. The message was to trust God with your life!!!! Imagine that – I just THOUGHT there was no way for God to send me a message. The message was not whether or not to have the lymph nodes radiated, but that no matter what happened, trust God with my LIFE. They offered the statement, "I trust you, God, with my life", and those seven words have kept me going in many difficult situations since. Imagine, me thinking God had no way to get to me!! You would have thought I would have learned by this time.

The Right Place, the Right Time for a Purpose

In the chapter on radiation, I mention that I was kept waiting for over half an hour on my first visit. At the time I was very upset and scared, but I came to realize that God had placed me in that specific situation for a reason. Without that time to sit and observe, I would not have seen other women and their reaction to wearing a hospital gown. Now there is a sign that a gown is not required and other options are available. If it had not been for that wait, I would not have seen this exchange – God wanted me there for a reason.

The Princess Speaks

A sign from the animal kingdom – or should I say – Queendom??? My loving kitty cat, Molly, is a true princess. I think she may have been royalty in another life, but either way, she is a sweet, loving cat in my life. She has graced my life for over 14 years, and in all that time she has slept in a lot of places, but never on my head!!! That is until the night before I went into the hospital for the partial mastectomy surgery. That night, and many nights since then, Molly slept right on my pillow snuggled in as close as possible to my head that she could get. I now call her my "Angel Kitty", because I truly believe she senses something was changing in my life, and she was there to help me in any way possible. Some people may be very skeptical about this idea, and that if fine, but for some of the true animal lovers reading this, I am sure you could share your own stories about how animals seem to have a keen sense of need, and I am so thankful that they do!

Passing it On

Even as I was writing this book, God continued to send me signs that there is a purpose for sharing with each other along this journey. Another dear friend of mine, Humor Team Member, and fellow clown, Linda, just recently shared a story with me about laughter and healing. Here was the message I received from Linda:

> "My long time friend Libby was diagnosed with breast cancer and I suggested a party. After she gasped, I told her Tammy's story. She reluctantly agreed to a few friends (a humor team) around her kitchen table. I told her Rosie (Linda's clown character) was coming, in plain clothes. We would be silly and laugh.
>
> In the few short weeks before this party, Libby started chemo. She was weakened and tired by Saturday. There have been no gatherings at Libby's house for years. She planned this kitchen table party near her bed/bath room "just in case." With Rosie in my shopping bag, I arrived at Libby's to discover twice as many people had been invited!
>
> Rosie was asked to perform. My small hospital experience quickly became a living room adventure.
>
> My most priceless picture is Libby looking absolutely beautiful. I hear her laughter and look to see she is smiling broadly with her colorful silk scarf wrapped around her almost bald head with a clown nose on. (I hope we have a picture!)."

Lesson Fourteen– *Know that you have choices. There are a lot of CHOICES that YOU can make. Keep in mind, the professionals are giving us options and choices. From there WE decide what we want to have happen to our body. This can only be determined from our own personal feelings, not our family, or friends, or strangers in the street. You were given a brain at birth, this is the time to engage the function of that brain and decide what is best for YOU! The caution here is to get all of the information you can find, so that you are thoroughly informed (see Lesson Ten).*

Chapter Fourteen
A Very Difficult Decision

"What is popular is not always right, and what is right is not always popular."
— Unknown Author

As many times as I have worked on this book over the last 2 years, I have stumbled on what to say in this chapter, but I believe this chapter may be the most important one in the book – maybe that is why it was so difficult to write.

When faced with a breast cancer diagnosis, there are many decisions to make, but I strongly believe we have to weigh all the options and make the right decision for ourselves. We are all different and we have to live with the decisions we make. The frustration I faced with one particular decision is that no one was ever going to tell me I had another option! Let's begin…

As I mentioned in a previous chapter, the decision of what to do about the breast was very involved, but I felt very comfortable about the decision I had made, and was pleased with the outcome.

Now it was time to make another decision involving chemotherapy. I really hated the idea of this process and I firmly believe it was putting poisons in my system – and in big doses. I am also one who is very easy to "toss my cookies" so I wasn't looking forward to that either. Most importantly, I still do not believe that this would have been a guarantee that I would not have to face this again, but it certainly was a standard procedure for a woman in my situation, with my diagnosis.

As I was researching the different types of chemo and the idea of having a shunt surgically implanted for ease of dispensing the chemo to the body, I came across another option.

(Before I go any further, let me put in a paragraph for Dr. B, Dr. W, and all the other healthcare people out there. I am not in any way, shape or form suggesting that my doctors did not know what they were talking about. In reality, I think I was truly blessed with the fantastic healthcare people I encountered during this journey, but I believe I had to be informed of more options than just the "standard" treatments. Thank you to all of you who allowed me to make my own decisions.)

I can say I "stumbled" on another option, but I truly believe I was "led" to another option by God. I pray each day that I made the right decision, but I go back to the strange feeling that I was led to it for a reason – a feeling that has been affirmed many times since. Sometimes the affirmations are in small things people say, other times they fall into the category of direct signs from God, as I mentioned in a previous chapter.

While searching the internet I noticed a couple of references to an "oopherectomy" (or ovarian ablation) as an alternative to chemotherapy for women fitting four very specific criteria, 1) pre-menopausal, 2) estrogen-receptor positive, 3) cancer of 2 cm or less, and 4) Stage I (if you are unfamiliar with this term, all cancers are "staged", with the stage being determined by how far the cancer has spread. For a more technical description, please refer to one of the books listed in the reference section). Since I fit <u>all four</u> criteria, the articles had my attention.

The theory behind this option is that if the cancer is estrogen-receptor positive (and you meet the other criteria) and you remove the producer of estrogen, the ovaries, then it can be just as effective as chemotherapy. Oopherectomy is just a medical term for the removal of the ovaries versus a hysterectomy that also removes the uterus.

When I had the name for this procedure, I was able to find quite a number of articles relating to this procedure, including an article from Johns Hopkins by Dr. Nancy Davidson, a Professor of Oncology, Johns Hopkins Oncology Center. Dr. Davidson had presented a paper on this procedure to a large medical conference the November before I was diagnosed.

The idea is not new, and in fact, doctors performing this procedure were awarded the Nobel Prize in the late 1800's in Sweden.

The situation was how to get MY doctors to look at the option. I had an appointment with Dr. W, an Oncologist in with Dr. B regarding when I should start the chemo. There is a time element involved in having chemo within 6-8 weeks after the surgery. Dr. W had to have some surgery himself (we forget that doctor's need this stuff sometimes, too) so it was very difficult to reach him with my questions. Fortunately, I was able to ask Dr. B some of the questions and he referred me to a nurse who worked with oncology and offered me a book to read about breast cancer treatments in general. I will not mention the title of the book or the nurse I spoke to, as they both became a great source of distress in my life.

I had read the chapter in the book about chemo and the different types of medication they mix for the chemo. The book stated that there was one particular kind that was more dangerous than the rest and had actually caused this doctor's patient to require a heart transplant! I was instantly scared and was fretting over what to ask Dr. W. I called the nurse that was recommended and asked her if she knew what Dr. W used for the chemotherapy mixture. You guessed it, the mixture I had just read bad reviews about. I asked her why he chose this mixture and her response was – are you ready for this???? Her response was, "He just does and you don't have a choice." Note the quotation marks – those were her exact words!! I decided at that point that I did not need to speak to this woman, and I did not need to read any more in that particular book. I DID have a choice – I could choose to die, if I wanted to. I was so furious with this woman, and in fact, I can clearly say this was the most angry I was during the entire journey! Remember, you ALWAYS have a choice, and I am sure this person did not realize how important the idea of choices is to a patient. Yes, we have to live with the ramifications of that choice, but there is always a choice. This exchange and the associated anger was clearly another part of that feeling out of control. When faced with this type of diagnosis, even the smallest amount of control can be vital to your life.

I calmed down a bit and contacted Dr. B. I think he could detect the stress in my voice, and since this was the first time he had truly heard it, he knew something wasn't right. I knew there was a time issue involved, and, with Dr. W being off for his surgery, I wasn't able to talk with anyone else. Dr. B was fantastic, as usual. He calmed me down and told me that he knew Dr. W very well, and there wasn't any chance of me having to have chemo until I had all my questions answered. Given the relationship we had developed, this immediately put my mind at rest. Dr. B was the one who would do the shunt, if I decided to go that route, and he made sure I realized we could work out the scheduling.

Before my appointment with Dr. W I did a ton of research on the oopherectomy. I had all the information I thought pertinent in a folder and was ready to explore this option. I dropped off an envelope to his office a few days before my appointment with a list of questions. (They are included in the chapter on questions.) I had used the NIH site and a few others and had all my questions outlined, as well as the report from Johns Hopkins. Armed with the stuffed folder, clown noses, and video camera, I was ready to meet with Dr. W.

Meeting Dr. W

Dr. W turned out to be a delightful man. He reminded me a lot in stature of Dr. B, and his bedside manner was very lighthearted and friendly – just my kind of person. This was to be one of the strangest meetings of the whole journey. You can think what you want and believe what you want, but I clearly believe there was something going on in that room that was spiritual in nature. When Dr. W came in he also had a folder of information. On the NIH website, you have a choice of information for patient or physician. I had all the patient information, and Dr. W came in with the physician information – I thought that was great!! I felt so empowered that I was involved in the decisions that were made in my life, and I was using a good source to do it.

    The conversation started, camera rolling, and we discussed the options of chemo, lymph node results, and the oopherectomy. Regarding the lymph nodes, although the initial test at the time of surgery indicated the lymph nodes were cancer free, the more involved test indicated there was a "trace" in one of the nodes. However, after we discussed the numbers, it was determined to be an insignificant amount on the scale, and I opted not to have the remaining lymph nodes removed. On the topic of the chemo vs. the oopherectomy, he said he was familiar with the idea, "But we just don't do it that way in the United States." We went back and forth and back and forth for about 10 minutes, and then the most amazing thing happened. He just stopped in mid-sentences and said, "Okay, maybe this is the best option for you." I swear to you, it was like a spirit was moving through the room and his whole attitude changed. I have this recorded on tape, and it is still apparent to me that there was a significant change taking place.

    Once we reached this point, he said he would do everything he could to help me have this alternate treatment. I asked him what we did next and he said he needed to find an expert on the topic and call the insurance company for approval. Well, I had the name and information of the "expert" in my folder. I handed it over to him and we were on our way.

A couple of days later he called me and said he contacted Johns Hopkins and talked with the "expert" there – found her very knowledgeable and good to talk with, but it is what he said during that conversation that was so important to me. He said, "Tammy, you have to understand we don't treat it this way in the United States, which is not to say it isn't the best treatment for you. After talking with Dr. Davidson, I believe this is the right treatment for you." I think I heard a faint sound of harp music somewhere!

Dr. W contacted the insurance company and got the approval for the procedure. I thought the hardest part was over – then I met Dr. C!! I didn't really have a gynecologist so I wasn't partial to any one person. We were still on the time line so I just needed a good doctor to do this surgery, and rather fast. Dr. W said he would help with that if I needed, but gave me a doctor's group to call.

Before I met the doctor, I told Dr. B what I was planning on doing. One of the greatest things about Dr. B was that he never said I was stupid or this was a bad decision, he simply was not very familiar with the procedure and why it was done in this case. He did suggest however, that since I had decided to go on Tamoxifen and a risk of Tamoxifen is uterine cancer and I was finished having children, I might consider a total hysterectomy. I thought this was very sound advice and decided that was the direction I was taking.

A side note to this decision affected the writing of this book. For the longest time I felt that I didn't have any "right" to write this book because I never really "suffered" like a lot of breast cancer patients and endured chemotherapy. This may sound crazy to you, but what I came to realize is that I NEEDED to write this book, and specifically this chapter because I DID choose a different treatment. One may not be any better than the other, but the key point is that it was a choice!

Exploring Alternatives

Before I go into the chapter about becoming a "Hyster Sister", I would like to address the issue of alternative treatments. I am not advocating in this chapter that you should ignore your doctor's advice, but I am advocating that you should embrace YOUR life and make informed decisions. There are a lot of treatments that are used to help not only cancer patients, but people facing various challenges in life.

While I was writing this book, a dear friend was diagnosed with breast cancer and ultimately decided on a double mastectomy, due in part because of her family history. One method of healing that she believes in is referred to as "healing touch". Not only has she studied and performs healing touch, but she also receives this method of healing. There are a number of different ways that healing touch can be performed, but basically it is a theory of using the body's own energy to help heal. I had a few healing touch sessions myself with my friend, and while I went into it a little skeptical, I did experience a sense of heat that I could not explain and it made a believer out of me that there was "something" going on with this type of healing.

After my surgeries, I went to see a woman who does this type of healing. I think the primary reason I went to see her was that she was a well respected friend of some friends and she was a survivor! She actually went so far as to go into the operating room with patients to help "heal" them as they were coming out of the surgery. The theory is that when anesthetic is put in our bodies, it can be toxic to the system for some people. The healing provided by this method quickly removes the anesthetic, builds the body's natural energy up more quickly, and the patient can start to heal immediately.

There are other programs out there designed to help people recovering from a variety of illnesses and these programs are gaining some important recognition. Ermyn King of Penn State University's Arts and Health Outreach Initiative (AHOI), a three-year interdisciplinary partnership pilot project devoted to demonstrating and documenting the interrelationships between the arts and health, has just concluded a three year program that established that significant interest exists within the University as well as nationally and internationally to explore the impact of the arts on personal and public health. The results of this initiative, which involved a wide variety of arts, including painting, music, dance, and, of course, clowning, just to name a few, has been highly successful to create other learning programs. The partnerships involved in this initiative are now taking the initiative to develop other programs of research, teaching and outreach that explore the areas of arts in healing, arts in human development, and the arts in community development.

    Another method of healing that is starting to draw a lot of attention in the news recently is the healing power of prayer. I even heard it mentioned in passing as possibly being the "next frontier" in healing. While people in the religious sect have long believed in this power, it is now gaining the attention of people in the sciences as a true method of helping to heal. From a scientific viewpoint, there is evidence to support that when a person prays, the body releases nitric oxide, a gas that aids in the healing for people with many illnesses. (There is even a Nitric Oxide Society out there for people to gain more insight into this phenomenon.) I am sure this particular information will be studied for years to come, but it is another idea that you can explore for your personal healing.

    Personally, I already know the power of prayer and have experienced it in my own life; not only on this journey, but on previous journeys as well. I firmly believe that the power of personal prayer and having people pray for my needs played a major role in my recovery!

    The idea of this section on alternative healing methods

is that there are countless ideas out there relating to treatment and healing. It may very well be difficult to discern the truth about all of the ideas, but I think you owe it to yourself to explore other options outside the "traditional" treatments, and then make your own decisions. I have had several doctors tell me on the course of this journey that there are "no guarantees" with any of treatments we use, and a lot of things that cannot be explained, both good and bad, so we all have to make the best decisions we can and take one day at a time.

Lesson Fifteen – *You are a unique person – there is no one else like you! Just because someone else experienced pain or problems, does not mean you will! The importance of this realization is that sometimes we set our minds up to expect pain or discomfort and we psychologically feel it because we mentally "expect" to. The same can be said for thinking the positive. In fact, that is a basic premise throughout this book. Set your mind to the positive – set your mind to recovery.*

Chapter Fifteen
Becoming a Hyster Sister

"Life is either a daring adventure or nothing at all."
— *Helen Keller*

It seems that women will bond over some of the funniest things! A cup of tea, a beautiful quilt, a good book, or maybe a hysterectomy??? As the relationship-oriented gender, we tend to depend on one another for friendship and support in all kinds of situations. While I didn't know it at the time, my hysterectomy would lead to one of those situations.

I set up an appointment and met Dr. C. I told her what I wanted and why I was there and she looked at me as though I was absolutely crazy! In fact, she would not agree to do this until I "thought about it" and came back again. She said she needed time to check out this procedure. She then said the funniest thing; she said she couldn't do the procedure because she was sworn "to do no harm". I just looked at her and asked if she thought chemo did no harm to the body!!! Either way, she wouldn't agree until she checked it out and I came back.

I made another appointment and went back again a week later. She said she had checked with some colleagues and they were divided on the treatment. She said she was concerned about me and my image as a woman – if all the "female" parts were removed. I truly don't think she realized either who she was talking to, or what she had said. Personally, I do NOT define myself as a woman simply by my "body parts"!! She wanted me to talk to the colleague who was uncertain about the procedure, but I noticed she didn't necessarily want me to talk to the colleague who thought the procedure was a viable option.

She actually made me come back a third time before she would agree to do the procedure and we finally set a date. I had contacted Dr. W before the third visit, and he told me that if she didn't agree to do it, not to worry, he would find someone who would do this procedure for me. Can you imagine – I thought it was going to be difficult to convince the oncologist and the insurance company and after that it would be smooth sailing. I kept telling myself I didn't have to "like" the doctor, she was just an end to a means! I made sure she had a good supply of clown noses and we left it at that.

What I did not know was that God had a plan – I love it when He does this!!!

The surgery was scheduled for almost 2 months after the major breast surgery, and a week before Christmas. Three surgeries in 2½ months – not something I wanted to do on a regular basis!!!

While I was waiting for the surgery date to arrive, I was doing research on hysterectomies. I know you're surprised, right? I found a really neat site on the internet at: www.hystersisters.com. I found the information offered to be informative, supportive and uplifting. The mission statement of this site is:

> Hystersisters.com is a woman to woman support website for hysterectomy recovery. It is not intended to take the place of a personal physician. The Hyster Sisters site is neither anti hysterectomy nor pro hysterectomy, rather, it is an online community of women who give and receive support for hysterectomy decisions and recovery. Hystersisters.com offers resources and kindness so that our visitors can discover options and make decisions for themselves.

If you find yourself in a similar situation or know someone dealing with this decision, you might want to check out the information offered by this site.

I arrived at the hospital at the appointed time and was armed with a fresh supply of clown noses AND a few other items to complete the ensemble!! The last time I was at the hospital for the breast surgery I was a little short of noses for all of the people in the operating room. They jokingly gave me a hard time about it, so this time I was armed with a big bag of noses and a sign that read, "I'm back with more noses for everyone, but I don't plan on coming back again, so this is all you get." This time I also had a feather boa, leopard Santa hat and matching leopard slippers – I was ready for action!

Dr. C came in and we had a nice little chat. I was compelled to tell her my feelings on the surgery and I think that broke the ice a bit. I told her that I truly believed that I was "led" to this option as an alternative to chemo, and I thought that she was chosen to be an instrument of God. It was an awesome responsibility, but I truly believed with my heart that it was the right decision, as difficult as it may have been to make.

She had a few deliveries going on and was going to put me in between a couple of Cesarean sections, so I might be ready early. That was fine with me and away we went to the operating room – BOA STILL AROUND MY NECK – INTACT!!! The surgery went well and when I woke up, the BOA WAS STILL IN PLACE!!! I understand she allowed me to wear it the whole time – hmm, part of the plan.

When I awoke in the recovery room, there was a party going on near my bed – AGAIN!!! It would seem that Dr. C decided she would not be out done by Dr. B and she had drawn a beautiful little clown face on the bandages covering my incision – hmm, another part of the plan! I wonder if all of these doctors are hidden artists?

The Chicken Comes to Life

After the surgery, I was sent to a room on the orthopedic floor because the OB-GYN floor was full – another fun part of the story. When I arrived at the room, I got out my bag of goodies and started looking for people to spring some humor on. One trick in my bag was a simple yellow towel. The gag with this towel is that it can be rolled and folded in such a way that you can create a rather life-like looking chicken. Of course there is a little music required from the participants to make it happen, but in all the time I have been doing "the chicken" I have never had a problem getting people to laugh. Although the gag came from a trip to Clown Camp, I don't know where the gag originated, but I thank whoever came up with the idea. I started with the nurses and my roommate and we had a nice laugh over the chicken. Since it was a big day for both me and my roommate, we decided to turn the lights off early and get some rest. Now, it might be important to remind you that I had had major surgery just a few hours before, and rest tends to be very beneficial to a quick recovery.

A couple of hours later I was sound asleep when a nurse came into the room. After all of these surgeries, by this time I was getting used to the idea of "wake up and take a sleeping pill", or some of the other crazy reasons that a sleeping patient is awaken at a hospital, but even this one floored me!! The nurse came into the room and shook me awake (honest!) and asked me to do "the chicken thing" for another nurse who had just come on duty!! I thought for a moment that I was still sleeping and was dreaming that I was in the office of Frank Purdue (the chicken guy), but quickly realized that was not the case. I pulled myself up in bed, got out the "chicken", started the request for music, created the chicken and collapsed back on the bed to go back to sleep. You know, you just can't make up this kind of stuff!!!

"Oh, What Did You Have Done?"

After the surgery I had really bad back pain, to the point that at midnight I rang for the nurse and asked if I could walk around. The response was "sure". Please remember here that I had MAJOR surgery less than 12 hours before, and the nurse simply got me up and let me roam the halls on my own. I was quite a distance from the Nurse's station and I thought it was a little odd to be left alone, but I didn't know any better.

After my extended walk, I went back to my room and a nurse stopped by to see if I needed something for pain. I said that I did, and while I was <u>standing</u> in my room, she put the pain medicine right in my IV and I almost passed out. I immediately got sick and thought I would faint. I am not a nurse, but I have been told since then that this is not a very good way to administer powerful medication! <u>After</u> I started to come around again, she actually looked at my chart and asked me what type of surgery I had and when it was. Hmm, in retrospect that may have been a good question to ask <u>before</u> allowing me out of bed alone, and before giving me the medication while I was standing!

Very early the next morning I was up and roaming the halls again. My attire was still the leopard print Santa hat with matching slippers, and my trusty feather boa. I passed the nurse's station and saw Dr. B sitting there working on charts. I said, "Good Morning, Dr. B." He took one look at me, laughed and shook his head and went back to the charts. I guess the strange outfits were now part of the "normal" routine. When I got back to my room, one of the nurse's came in and said a patient had just stopped her and asked if there was someone roaming around the halls wearing a feather boa, or if she was just seeing things. We both had a good laugh!

The following morning an associate of Dr. C's came to see me and when he found out what had happened during the night, he quickly arranged to have me moved to the OB-GYN floor. It was indeed an exciting night though and made for a good story!

Another Plan Comes Together!

My recovery went extremely well and Dr. C was amazed at how quickly I recovered. The most touching moment of the whole story happened on the morning I was to be discharged. Dr. C came to visit about 7:00 AM. Like most people, I was anxious to get OUT of that hospital, and since this was the third surgery in just over two months, I had had quite enough! Dr. C sat down beside my bed and we softly chatted about how I was feeling and how things were going. I introduced her to "the chicken" and we shared a good laugh. After she checked all the vital signs and went over the discharge information, she said something that I will never forget. We had both had a rough start to this patient/doctor relationship, but she leaned over and said, "You have taught me so much. I feel that I am now better able to care for my other patients." Obviously, I don't think I taught her much, but God used me to teach her. I love it when a plan comes together!!!

The Chicken Lives Again

Dr. C had given me a prescription for pain that I was to have filled before going home that morning. When I stopped at the pharmacy to have it filled, there was a problem with the dosage and I was unable to get it filled as written. We went to a couple of different places, and finally realized that the dosage was not common in our area and I would need to have another prescription written and filled. A quick phone call to Dr. C's office took care of the problem and we headed to her office for a new prescription and to have it filled at the pharmacy in her office area.

The reason I am telling you this is that it took a little while to get a prescription filled for pain after I had left the hospital. With the discharge procedure and getting ready to go, there was quite a while between pain medications and the pain was getting quite intense. When I walked into the doctor's office to get the new prescription I was asked to wait for just a couple of minutes until the nurse could get to me. No problem, quite a bit of pain, but I knew the medication was in sight to give me some relief. What I did not know was that there was going to be another crazy delay!

When I was finally called back to the doctor's office to get the prescription, the nurse met me at the desk with a prescription AND, did you guess it, A TOWEL!!! She said she didn't know exactly what I was to do with it, but Dr. C told her I would know what to do! I am sure I gave her a really strange look (maybe it was really a grimace in pain) before I cracked up laughing and started the chicken! She didn't have a yellow towel handy, but she did have a white one, so we had a chicken of white meat. I laughed and laughed, which wasn't easy to do with fresh stitches from a hysterectomy, but I finished the chicken, grabbed the prescription and got out of there! CJ was sitting out in the waiting room and could hear this whole exchange. When I came out he just looked at me and said, "Did they ask you to do what I think they did?" Yes, you guessed it, the chicken lives!

A Truly Wild Woman

As you may have gathered from the earlier exchange with Dr. C, I found her to be a rather conservative person. I certainly grew to like her a great deal, even though the beginning wasn't the smoothest, but I still thought she was a little conservative.

When I went in for my two week check-up, I came armed with a bag of gratitude goodies for Dr. C that included her very own feather boa. She thanked me and seemed to blush as she opened the small package.

When it was time to go in for my six week check-up after the surgery, I had to wait for a little while in the examination room. It wasn't a long wait, but her nurse said Dr. C may be just a bit longer than usual. No problem, I was catching up on the latest magazine when the door literally "burst" open, and my seemingly conservative Dr. C came through the door with her clown nose on and feather boa blowing in the breeze she had just created!! We both had a wonderful laugh and I knew there was hope for Dr. C!!!

Lesson Sixteen – *Celebrate even the smallest victories. As you have read, I am a big one for celebrating the smallest victories. Maybe I am just a party animal, but when you are dealing with a life-changing situation, whatever that situation may be, there are times when you feel you have to find something good in the situation. Celebrate something, anything at least once a week. Each day is a gift and gifts are meant for parties. Maybe you have to use your imagination a little stronger on some days, but don't forget to celebrate.*

Chapter Sixteen
Another Very Special Party

"Every once in a while life hands you a moment so precious, so overwhelming, that you almost glow."
— *Unknown Author*

I have said before that I am always looking for a reason for a good party, okay, so I don't REALLY need a reason, but on this journey, there was another very special party that I didn't even attend!

I belong to an organization called Toastmasters International. In the most simplistic terms, it is a wonderful group of people who meet in a "club" atmosphere to help each other build communication skills. (I wouldn't be doing my part for the organization if I didn't put in a little commercial here. Check it out at www.toastmasters.org. It might just change your life. It certainly did mine!)

Each year our local clubs get together in December and have a holiday party. It is always a lot of fun and we have a great time sharing a meal, good conversation and a rather unusual gift exchange. I have to take a moment to explain this gift exchange so you get the full impact of this very special party.

Each person attending the party brings a wrapped gift, the zanier the better, and we all draw numbers from a hat. The person with number one goes first and takes a gift, removes the wrapping and places it in front of him/her. The person with number two takes a gift, removes the wrapping then gives a one to two minute mini-speech about why they are going to keep the gift they have chosen, or exchange it for the gift chosen by the person with the number one. This continues for the entire group, then finally the person with the number one gets to choose the last gift and decide if they want that one or any of the other gifts that have been chosen throughout the evening. It is really a great deal of fun, and usually there are a few gifts that change hands many, many times around the room.

    I was unable to attend this particular party as I was home recuperating from the hysterectomy. It is always a highlight of the holiday season, so I was very disappointed that I could not attend. What I did not know is that a very special Toastmaster friend, Bruce, had worked it out with CJ and the rest of the Toastmasters group to do a special honorary party for me this year. The premise was changed to respond to the question, "What is the craziest gift at the party, and why would it be perfect for Tammy?" The whole party was taped, and some of the tributes from the people responding about the gifts brought me to tears. It was so moving and touching, that my eyes mist over just remembering the event as I write this section.

    The gift that ultimately came home to me was a huge bumblebee – the perfect gift. Remember, as a clown, the idea of a "perfect gift" may not seem like the norm for other people. You just never know when you might need an over-sized bumblebee!! Bumblebee or not, gift or no gift, the true gift was the deep thoughtfulness of my friends at the party, and this certainly helped aid my recovery!

Yet Another Special Group of People

    As I mentioned before, one of my jobs is at a major university. As part of the benefits package, if there is a serious illness and you use all of your allotted sick days, you can ask for a "vacation donation" of up to 30 days from your co-workers, but each employee is limited to donating one day. As much as I hated to do it, I needed some extra time to recover from the hysterectomy and probably the whole ordeal so I asked for the possibility of a vacation donation. I am told that when the message went out from the Human Resources department, the replies came in so quickly from my fellow employees that the 30 day allotment was filled within two hours! It turned out that I didn't need to take the entire 30 days, but what a wonderful blessing to know there were so many people who cared!

Lesson Seventeen – *Accept that there are some things in life we cannot change. Learning to look for the brightest spots can make a tremendous difference! Look for them, celebrate them, they are everywhere! Sometimes learning how to determine what we can and cannot change is the hardest lesson of all.*

This goes back to the *Serenity Prayer* that was penned long ago:

God grant me the serenity

to accept the things I cannot change;

courage to change the things I can;

and wisdom to know the difference.

When we are faced with something that spins our life out of control, sometimes the fine line of control gets a little gray. Look for what you can change and start there. Even the smallest circumstances (and they are everywhere), can make a difference.

Chapter Seventeen
A Few "Normal" Responses –
Please Define "Normal"

"A great opportunity is often described as an impossible situation." — Unknown

As I mentioned before, this journey has certainly been an adventure! In the chapter on "Waiting" I described a series of "days" that I seemed to have experienced that involved everything from uproarious laughter, to REALLY crazy thoughts, to varying levels of apprehension and concern. In this chapter I would like to reinforce the idea that there is no "normal" response to a breast cancer diagnosis, or any serious medical concern or challenge in life. We are all unique individuals and there isn't a textbook that could be written to tell us how we are suppose to respond in these situations.

Each of us will have different experiences on our personal journey, and it is vitally important to embrace the differences, whether they are happiness, sadness, frustration, or celebration. It is only when we learn to look to these aspects of our journey as lessons, that we can fully understand the true idea that "normal" is just a word on a page, but it is really no such part of life.

Choosing Your Battles

One of the great lessons I learned along this journey, and perhaps it really should be Lesson 21, is that we must choose our "battles" wisely. There were a couple of incidents on this journey that reinforced the idea that we are all given only so much energy. Often, misplaced energy doesn't benefit anyone and we have to examine not only how we will respond, but if it is worth the extra energy to really get upset.

The first test of this lesson came about five weeks after I have the partial mastectomy. You certainly know by this time in the book that I am persistent when it comes to medical appointments and if I hadn't been with the mammogram, the outcome may have been different. So that you have a timeline review, my surgical biopsy was October 8 (with preparation work being done at the Breast Care Center); and the partial mastectomy was October 25. In early December I received a letter from the Breast Care Center stating that "my recent mammogram has shown abnormalities but I had not taken action on this information". The letter then continued to state that "this could be very serious and I was urged to follow-up immediately with my doctor". I can tell you I was less than happy when I read the letter – still wearing small bandages to cover my incision.

I was very upset and wondered how in the world they could possibly make this mistake. It took a little while, but I realized that it was simply a mistake, and although it certainly wasn't good for the image of the Breast Care Center, the best that I could do was to bring this to their attention and hope that the next person would not have to deal with the same situation.

The second issue was one that I may never know the answer to. I still wonder if the cancer was missed on the mammogram the year before. I have had a couple of people look at it, and they are just not sure. Obviously, I am not a trained professional, but I have always wondered how it could have grown so quickly to get to the 2 cm size in the time between the mammograms. Again, I expended some energy on this, but came to realize that there wasn't anything I could do to change it, even if it was missed, and I needed all the positive energy I could gather to heal and recover, so in the entire scheme of life – it just didn't make a difference.

Afraid to Eat

During the time between the hysterectomy surgery and the radiation started, there were a lot of thoughts going through my mind. Perhaps, it would be better to say the thoughts were "racing" through my mind. I am not one to just sit still, as most of my family and friends would attest to, so sitting and actually "recovering" was difficult to do.

The decision about having the hysterectomy vs. the chemotherapy was already done and I was feeling very good about the decision. I had started the Tamoxifen and was having tremendous hot flashes from the medication. Even though the hysterectomy alone can certainly bring on hot flashes, I knew it was a reaction to the Tamoxifen as the "flashes" did not become intense until I started taking this medication. (As a side note, I have come to live with these "flashes" and think of them as a part of my total recovery. Since I do have them and expect to until I stop the Tamoxifen, I have come to call them my "energy surges". For some reason, calling them a surge just mentally feels better and seems to give me more "energy"! I am still working on ways to "bring them on" at the RIGHT time, for example, when it is very cold outside, but I haven't quite perfected that plan, yet.

Since the surges were so strong, I was not sleeping at all and I finally went back to Dr. C for a mild medication to help with the surges. There is some research indicating that very low doses of anti-depressant medications like Effexor can help women cope with intense surges. I took this medication for while and it did seem to take the edge off enough to let me sleep at nights. If you are bothered by intense hot flashes or "energy surges", you may want to discuss this option with your doctor. I also discovered certain "triggers" like caffeine and wearing polyester clothing would add to the intensity of the surge. If this is a problem for you and alters your lifestyle, you may want to pay closer attention to your personal surge triggers.

Since I wasn't sleeping, some of the smallest things seemed to bother me. I am sure I almost wore my mantra out as I was going through this period. Part of the reading that I was doing was about alternate methods to help with the hot flashes. Since my cancer was estrogen receptor positive, which basically meant it was feeding on estrogen, I would never be a candidate for hormone-replacement therapy. As part of the reading though, I came across the idea that many foods create a natural estrogen, for example, one of my favorites, broccoli. (Keep in mind that I was VERY tired!) When I read this, I had a panic attack about what other foods would create estrogen and would that estrogen bring the cancer back. I was so concerned that I actually stopped eating everything for a couple of days!! Now, not only was I VERY tired, but also VERY hungry!

My friend, Mary, stopped by to see me one afternoon. I didn't realize just how tired and hungry I was until she asked me how I was doing. In most cases this would be a simple question of caring and concern. In this particular case, it was an opening for the flood gates. I started to cry and cry and cry and I could not stop. Poor Mary wasn't exactly sure what was going on and between sobs I was trying to tell her I couldn't eat. Since I have never had a problem with my appetite in the past (bring on the chocolate anytime!), Mary was really confused about the reason behind the tears. I finally calmed down enough to give her the whole story and we talked for quite a while about this being another part of a "normal response" - confusion.

Our conversation calmed me considerably and I agreed to talk to the doctor about this, eat, and get some sleep, not necessarily in that order!

The next time I was in to see Dr. C, I discussed this issue and she offered the idea that the estrogen in natural foods is of a different chemical design than synthetic estrogen, and since Tamoxifen is an anti-estrogen drug, I needed to weigh the benefits I received from good, healthy foods and continue to eat in a healthy manner.

I left her office feeling better about broccoli and with a prescription for a low dosage medication to help with the surges. After a few days, I was finally able to get back on a routine of healthy eating and getting sleep.

In retrospect, the intensity of the emotions about eating was surprisingly strong. I believe it was still another reminder that there were and are no "normal" responses to a breast cancer diagnosis. We all have to find our own level of "normal".

Lesson Eighteen - *Keep your doctor and health care providers accountable to you. This is your health and your life. Don't waste each other's time, but make sure your doctor answers all of your questions, no matter how simple or complex. In the entire scheme of things, you see these people for a brief time over your lifetime. I am VERY thankful for the wonderful healthcare providers I met, but when the treatments are done, you have to live your life.*

Chapter Eighteen
When I am Radiated, I Shall Wear Purple, or Blue, or Plaid, or Red!

Those who make us laugh are many... Those who make our hearts smile are our friends...
— *Unknown Author*

What can I say about the whole radiation thing? Oh, yeah, the best thing to say is that those people are "NUTS"!! Since this was part of the healing and recovery process, and I had agreed to the treatment, I also had a choice as to how I would respond to the process of the treatments. I can tell you that I had the best group of people helping me through it that I could imagine. It didn't start out that way, but I very quickly realized that this was indeed a special team of people.

Gown? No, Thank You, I Brought My Own

The first stop in the hospital in preparation for the radiation was to have a CT scan done to examine the breast. The CT scan is a way to look at a cross section of the body, producing more detailed results than a normal x-ray can produce. Since I had already gone through three surgeries in just over 2½ months, I had developed a real dislike for hospital gowns. In fact, I had stopped wearing them on my visits to the doctors, and instead just made sure I wore tops that could be unbuttoned in the front and easily removed if necessary. From a patient's perspective, you are already in an uncomfortable place; often times scared, and you are asked to remove a personal piece of your dignity so that it is easier for someone else. Please understand, when it is a situation of sterilization, that's different, but I had come to discover that most of these situations were not a matter of cleanliness, and I wasn't about to give up that tiny, personal piece of "control" (there's that word again!).

The first thing the technician asked me to do was to get into a gown. I had brought along two different pieces of clothing from home with all intentions to wear one of those instead. After the initial shock that I wasn't just going to put the gown on, it was determined that what I brought really wasn't good for the test because one material contained tiny pieces of metal and the other had buttons. Okay, okay, just this once! One of the therapists from the Radiology Department, Toni, was also in the room, and I found out later that she was very concerned that day that I was going to be a "real pain" of a patient, due in part because of the "problem" I gave them about not wearing a gown. (Thankfully, we had a good laugh about it later – much later – the end of my treatments!)

When I actually arrived at the Radiology department I was very upset and nervous. I don't think it was anxiety about the radiation. I had started Tamoxifen on January first and it was making the nightly hot flashes so intense I could not sleep more than one or two hours at a time. My appointment in Radiology was on the 17th of January so I had not slept well for almost three weeks by this point. The lack of sleep was starting to take its toll.

When I arrived, I was asked to sit in the waiting room and wait for the nurse. I was truly upset by what I saw. The room was about 10 feet by 10 feet with chairs lining the walls, a television suspended from the ceiling, a small refrigerator, and a coffee station. In other words, the room was slightly crowded. The thing that upset me was that the women there for treatments were sitting in this room with hospital gowns, some very poorly fitting, while CJ and I were fully dressed and in street clothes. I felt that this was a slap at personal dignity. Was it really necessary to wear a hospital gown for these treatments? Did they have to seat the people in gowns with "the public"?

There were four women in gowns, but one that really shook my foundation. This woman, in her late fifties, came in and sat down. She had already changed into her gown, but it was her behavior that still haunts me. She must have been going through chemo at the same time, or had shortly finished, as she didn't have any hair on her head. Instead, she had a poorly made wig, almost like a piece of fur stuck to her head. She was a very large busted woman, and the entire time she was there she kept pulling the gown up around her neck and my heart just went out to her. I had already decided that I would NOT be wearing a gown during my visits, but more on that in a minute.

The nurse ushered us into the examination room after waiting for a half hour. She proceeded to ask all kinds of questions as expected, but what I was upset about is the fact that I had recently had two surgeries in this hospital – just a few feet away. The answers to all of her questions were already in a file. I had even called ahead of time and asked if the file could be retrieved from the records area, but this had not been done. So we went through the questions once again.

I must admit, I was not in the best of moods and I let the nurse know I was upset. I stopped, took a couple of deep breaths, and apologized for my outburst. I truly know it wasn't her fault, but I really dislike inefficiency in any area. I also think I would have felt much better about the situation if I had not been kept waiting for a half hour, and if I would have had just a little sleep. That sleep depravation thing can really be a bear! She then gave me a gown to put on and I pulled my own out of the bag and told her I would not be needing one, thank you, I had brought my own! I am sure from her response that no one had ever done that before, but then again, I wasn't anyone's usual patient!

While I was waiting for the doctor I was reading through a booklet that I had picked up in the waiting room. It was again nice to see that the information I had gathered from my internet search was some of the same information offered in this book. The booklet was published by the National Institutes of Health, National Cancer Institute. The title was *Radiation Therapy and You: A Guide to Self-Help During Cancer Treatment.* More information can be found regarding this booklet in the reference section at the back of this book.

Dr. D introduced himself and my immediate impression was "all business". (I certainly came to see that, like the others, Dr. D had a very caring and sweet demeanor.) After the basic questions and answers, I started with a few more technical questions that I had formulated from a scientific article I had read. It dealt with the type of rays that were used during the radiation and what can be done to protect the heart. In reality I don't think I have a scientific bone in my body, but I must have sounded believable because Dr. D's whole body language changed as he realized that I had done some homework and was taking a great interest in my personal treatment. I don't know how many people he gets who come "armed" with questions, but in my quest for that little bit of "control" again, I was ready! He answered all of my questions at a level that I could understand and I was satisfied with the outcome.

If you are inclined to look for some more of the technical information on radiation therapy, there are a number of sites available. One site I would recommend is the Radiation and Oncology journal on line. The web site address to get you started is: www.elsevier.com/locate/radonline.

At the end of our meeting, I told him I didn't plan on wearing a hospital gown on any of my visits for the next seven weeks. I assured him my clothes would be metal free and clean; did he see a problem with that? He smiled and said he didn't think it would be a problem. (I wore all kinds of brightly colored shirts for the treatments, but more about that a little later.) Woo-hoo – another little victory!!

The Treatments

The duration and strength of the radiation one receives is determined by the size, location, and stage of the cancer. For me, it was determined that I would have 34 treatments – five days a week, Monday through Friday for almost 7 weeks. I would also have to make a decision whether or not I wanted the associated lymph nodes radiated. In the chapter titled "Signs from God" this was one of the decisions that I wrestled a great deal with before I was confident of my decision. However, once the decision was made and the treatments were done, I knew in my heart it had been the right decision.

After the initial consultation, my first real appointment was to have something called a "simulation" done in Radiology. This process is basically to determine EXACTLY where on the breast the radiation treatments would be given. What I remember best about this session was that the room was FREEZING!!! Dr. D and his assistant, Susan were taking all kinds of pictures and making all kinds of markings on my breast. They kept telling me to hold still, and I finally told them that if they wanted me to hold still, they were going to have to turn up the heat, because my bones were chattering!!! That was the first of many laughs in Radiology!

By the time they were done, my breast looked like a play book for the "big game". This was all done in permanent marker and different colors so that it would not have to be repeated on subsequent visits. These markings were what they would use to line up the radiation beams and they would stay in place until I received my "tattoos". (I wondered if I would get to choose the colors and designs for my tattoo – maybe a nice little flower....)

Meeting the Gang!

Although I saw the doctor and nurses often, and everyone was really great, it was the team of three radiation therapists that I saw the most and with whom developed the closest bond. Chris, Toni, and Susan became the "Morning Team"!!! I had already passed out clown noses to some of the people I had met, but I decided it was time to go beyond the nose and really embrace the situation.

The procedure was for me to come to Radiology every morning at 8:00 AM, change into "my" gown, sit in the waiting room until called, and then go back to the treatment room for the treatment.

The treatment itself really only lasted about 5 to10 minutes and was <u>absolutely painless</u>. It took longer for them to position me on the table than it did for the treatment. The most memorable part of the treatments was that there was a series of five "noises" as they repositioned the machine. Throughout the entire seven weeks, I felt very little sensation from the treatments. On a couple of days I felt a brief "tingling", but that was all from the actual treatments.

Gotcha'!

The day after the first real treatment, I decided to let the staff know that we were in this together for the long haul. Remember the "Sculpty" nipple? Well, it was time to get it back out again.

I used the latex adhesive and positioned the nipple on my upper stomach, close to the chest. It looked like a third nipple between where the "real" nipples are – okay, between where the right nipple is and the left nipple used to be – detail, details.

When I came through the door for my treatment, Chris and Toni were waiting for me. I burst through the doors saying, "I don't know what happened, but I had some sort of reaction to the treatment!" Both of them looked at me with concern and asked what the problem was, expecting rash, sores, or something terrible. I just opened my shirt and said, 'I don't know, but I don't think this is normal!" It took them a split second, and then they both burst out in laughter. One of them mumbled something about putting a sanity check on my chart, but we went on from there.

After the treatment, they had to bring Susan in and show her, and then they set the nurse, Joanie, up for the gag. Poor Joanie, she was so concerned when they said there was a reaction, and I think she was speechless as she viewed the "problem". I think she was truly concerned about me, but I don't think it had to do with radiation, more likely my mental state!

Since this was a Friday and Dr. D was not in, they persuaded me to wear it again on Monday. Of course I did as instructed. When Dr. D took a look at it, he too was at a loss for words – at least the kind he could utter in public, and became concerned about my mental state. All in all, it was a great success, and I think it helped set the stage for the following few weeks.

On a serious note, I have mentioned this many, many times throughout the book, that I know I cannot change the diagnosis, but I am in control of how I respond. The people in the Radiation/Oncology department were there to help me recover, and if we could do that and have a fun time, then that was even better.

The whole nipple incident must have made an impact. A week later I e-mailed Dr. B just to give him an update on my progress and he e-mailed me back with a single line – "I hear you cracked them up in Radiation". Hmm, all these people talking about my nipples!! What a riot!!

A Tattooed Woman

I mentioned earlier that the markings from the "simulation" had to stay on my chest until I received my tattoos. The thought of receiving a PERMANENT tattoo was very upsetting to me. I had never been one to want a tattoo on my body, and in this case it would serve as a constant reminder that I had had cancer – no thank you – or at least that is how it started.

During my initial consultation with Dr. D we briefly discussed the tattooing. He said it was very tiny, but I still didn't want anything to do with it. He went so far as to have Chris come in and "show" me a tattoo mark that he had put on his hand to show the size that I would receive. I didn't really know Chris yet, and he couldn't even find the tattoo, so I wasn't sure I believed any of this!

A couple of days after the treatments started it was time to have the tattoos done on my chest. The alternative to tattoos was to have the area re-marked on a regular basis and there was greater chance of error as the re-markings were done. With the tattoos, there was a marking point to line the machine up each time, and since they were permanent, it would be consistent.

In my case, I needed to have three tattoos. Even though I understood the need, I was especially upset that one of the marks had to be outside of what would be considered the "bra area".

I was really wrestling with the idea, but Chris and Toni were absolutely fantastic about the whole thing. We decided to compromise. Even though they told me the marks would be VERY tiny, I didn't know them very well yet and didn't quite trust their definition of "tiny". The compromise was that they would do two and I was to go home and wash off all of the other markings. If I was still upset about the tattoos, they would not do the upper one and we would just remark that one each time the marker wore off. This may sound petty to some, but this compromise was very important to me in that it was another little piece of "control" that I had in the decision making.

As it turned out, Toni is the one who did the tattoos, and I can honestly tell you they are VERY tiny. Toni told me that she always tried to make them exceptionally tiny because she felt that if she ever had to have this done, she would want very tiny marks. The day after I washed off the marking, the remaining tattoo was done and I have never been hesitant about the decision.

To give you an idea of the size of the tattoos I am talking about, if you would take a ball point pen and firmly touch it to your skin, it would probably be larger than the tattoos I now have on my breast and chest. The idea of a tattoo can still be a scary thought to some women. In fact, a close friend of mine was in tears as we discussed the idea of having a permanent tattoo until I showed her how small they actually are on the body. If you have to have this done, and it is a bothersome decision, be adamant about wanting it as small as they can possibly make it, and I wish you the skill and compassion of my team!

"Machine Down" Activities

As with most complicated equipment, every now and then there is a machine problem and you have to wait until someone comes in to fix the equipment. There were a couple of those days in Radiology, so we had to find our own entertainment while we were waiting for repairs.

The first time it was down, I had brought my camera and took pictures of the team. We joked that it was my turn to "take the pictures"!

The next time there were a few people in the waiting room and we were all disappointed that we would not be able to receive a treatment that day. There are been three or fours days in a row where the equipment was questionable and keep in mind, that each treatment got us closer to being done, so each delay meant another day at the end of the sessions.

On this particular day, I decided we all needed a break! I went to the car and brought in a supply of kazoos, stickers and my old faithful – the chicken towel!! The first Radiology Kazoo Band was born!!! The staff and patients all joined in "kazooing" and we had a great time passing the time. There was one older gentleman who was often in the waiting room at the same time that I was. After some brief instruction on the kazoo, he joined with the music and actually took the lead on a couple of songs! We shared kazoos, laughter, clown noses, and healing that day!

The following day I was greeted by the team playing their own kazoo rendition of "Grey Skies Are Going to Clear Up!"

Feeling Just Ducky

It was immediately obvious that my morning team had a great sense of humor, albeit twisted at times!!!

On one occasion I came around the corner into the treatment room singing, "She'll be Coming 'Round the Mountain". I looked up and Susan and Toni had taken gum pieces and made "beaver teeth" over their own. When I started singing this particular song, they cracked up and we all had a great laugh.

Not only were the colorful shirts getting attention from others, but the other patients started to refer to me as "the sock lady". It became a daily challenge to wear the craziest socks I could find to each treatment. I had yellow rubber duckies taking a bath on my socks one day. When I went in for the treatment, Susan said I looked really "Ducky", followed by Toni's, "Wait 'til she gets the bill", and Chris' usual smart remarks. They were just quacking me up – well, you can see where this was going!!!

They were also always complimenting my breasts. You know, with statements like, "That looks really good". Okay, so maybe they were talking about how the skin was responding to the treatments, but I will take any compliments I can get!

A Quick Comment on Burning

One of the primary concerns about receiving radiation is burning of your skin. For some, this is a minor problem, like a bad sunburn, and for others, there is severe discomfort. On the first day of the treatments, I was given a lotion to apply to the radiated area immediately following the treatment each day. The idea was to keep the area from burning. For the first six weeks I did not have any trouble at all, but then I changed my shampoo. One suggestion I have for anyone receiving this type of treatment is to be sure to keep using the same soaps and shampoos throughout the entire time. The same day I used a new shampoo, and the shampoo ran down across my chest, I burned with the treatment. I found out the hard way that a tiny little change could make a difference. The burn didn't last long and actually faded to a lovely golden brown, so if there is a brighter side, you know me, I have to try and find it!

The Boost

The last eight treatments I received are referred to as "the boost". Simply put, it is a different type of beam (electron) directed at the specific spot where the cancer was removed. Instead of five different "noises" from the machine, it was only one and it was administered through a cone-shaped instrument attached to the radiation head.

To get the proper measurement, there is a metal piece designed and cut specifically to radiate my body. It was a beautiful silver metal piece with my name on it. I asked if I could take it home and use it as a planter, but there was some comment made about toxic materials, so I decided to find something else for my pansies.

Since I had gone a couple of days without anything exciting happening, the day after my first boost it was time to liven the place up again. You remember my "Dolly Parton" wig? Well, it was time to bring it out again.

The radiation machine was not working properly on the first scheduled day of the "boost", and they weren't sure if it would be running on the second day. Finally, after a little wait I was able to get my first boost. I had my first boost on a Tuesday afternoon, and on Wednesday morning I got up a bit earlier and adjusted the full – I mean really full – head of golden curls.

There was a camera in the waiting room so the staff could see who was waiting when they were ready to call people back for a treatment. I decided I didn't want any of the therapists to see me in the waiting room so I would have to barge on in and greet them this morning.

As it turned out, the person who usually came in for a treatment ahead of me was not in that day, so as I walked through the door, the entire group was standing at the desk going over charts. As I walked through the door I said, "I don't know what you did to that machine, but I think that "boost" was a little strong. This is how I woke up this morning!!" What a riot!!! We all laughed until we hurt about the huge curls, and they had to take pictures for my file. Chris diagnosed the problem as "Post Boost Syndrome" and we had a really great laugh to start the day.

The boost signified a couple of things. First, the treatments were almost over, meaning I was well on the path to getting on with my life as a fully recovered cancer survivor. The second was actually very depressing. The end of the boost also signified the end of my morning "party" with the team in Radiation. I was really going to miss these people that had been an intricate part of my recovery team, especially Chris, Toni and Susan, since I worked closest with them. I found myself almost in a mild depression – we really had a lot of fun, but it was time to move on, but there was still time for another PARTY!

My Little Legacy

The very first morning I came into the treatment room I was wearing a bright blue oversized shirt and matching socks. It was actually just a man's shirt that I had borrowed from CJ (thankfully he likes bright colors!). It had buttons down the front and I simply put it on over my pants. After the initial surprise that I was not wearing a gown, "my team" embraced the idea of seeing brighter colors in the treatment room. The shirt was a PERFECT alternative to the hospital gown and just the feeling of wearing my own clothes made a tremendous difference in my attitude over the next seven weeks!

In fact, on many days while I was briefly seated in the waiting room, other women would make comment about the shirt vs. a gown and I encouraged them to try it as a colorful alternative. I am personally very proud to say that I left a sort of legacy in the Radiation department. Before my treatments were completed, the staff hung a sign that read:

To Our Patients

If you have been asked to change into a hospital gown for your treatments and do not feel comfortable in doing so, "please" speak with your therapist or nurse about other options available to you for your complete privacy and consideration.

Thank you!

I had talked with a co-worker who had received radiation four years earlier and she said the worse part about the entire ordeal was the terrible embarrassment she felt in the hospital gown while she waited. Maybe this will start a new trend everywhere. It certainly is a simple, colorful alternative!

(I stopped by the Radiology department while I was writing this book, and they are now offering very nice robes for the patients to wear. They are a white wrap-type robe with a colorful hospital logo embroidered on. I am not sure if there are plenty of size variations for everyone, but at least it is a start. I am still an advocate for colorful shirts that you know will fit you, but even the smallest changes can make a difference.)

Daffodils to Brighten the Day

While I was undergoing the treatments I received a bunch of daffodils at home one day. It turned out that Dr. B sent daffodils for the American Cancer Society Daffodil Days to all of his patients – what a sweet thought. The daffodils certainly brightened my day. (As a side note, with the new privacy laws, he is no longer allowed to do this – HIPPA strikes again. Hmmm, maybe getting that changed is a "battle" worth expending some of my energy!)

New Found Friends

The last day of my treatments was bittersweet. This part of my healing journey was over, but so were the smiling starts to each morning. My team certainly kept things lively and I will always cherish the time we spent together.

On the last day I brought little gifts (WILD SOCKS!!!) for each of my team members, and they actually surprised me with a gift. They gave me a beautiful little candle set and a lovely magnet that said:

> Those who make us laugh are many...
> Those who make our hearts smile are our friends.

I have the magnet hanging in my office where I see it everyday and think of the wonderful times shared with my "Morning Team".

While this part of the journey certainly didn't start out on a positive note, the friendships forged turned out to be one of the best parts of the journey.

Lesson Nineteen – *Thank your healthcare providers. Almost everyone I met along the path was very kind and considerate. They went out of their way to make me feel reassured when I was scared and comfortable when a procedure was difficult. Even though this may be "their job", it was the personal touch that made such a difference – that is not taught in a textbook. Whenever possible, thank them for being there to take care of you.*

Chapter Nineteen
THE RAG PARTY!!

"Gratitude is not only the greatest of virtues, but the parent of all others." — Cicero

At the end of the radiation treatments it was time for my Humor Team to throw another party!!! (What did you expect?) This time it was called the RAG Party. RAG stood for Random Acts of Gratefulness. The invitation read like this:

> As members in good standing of Tammy's
> Humor and Recovery Team,
> You are all cordially invited to attend a
>
> RAG Party
> (Random Acts of Gratefulness!!)
> Celebrating Tammy's
> Treatment Completion!!
>
> NOTES: EVERYONE should bring a rag with a story
>
> IF (not necessary) you want to bring a dish - food is limited to dishes that start with an R or A or G (hey, you can be very creative with "Appetizers" or "Rice", etc.)
>
> Come and join in the laughter and FUN!
> WIth good food and great conversation!!

Linda and Jerry once again hosted and people from the Radiology department attended with my Humor Team. Activities included a RAG Word Search that included the following words: boa, boobies, caring, doctor, feathers, gratitude, laughter, lopsided, love Mickey Mouse, party, red noses and treatments (not a complete list!).

And, there was another song!! This time it was to the tune of "Somewhere Over the Rainbow", but was re-titled, "She's Over the Rainbow". The lyrics were as follows:

> Now that you're over the rainbow
> and the treatments are thru,
> There's a nipple waiting for you
> comes in green, yellow, red, or blue.
>
> Here we join to celebrate it
> your new look.
> You've become nice and radiated
> Can we use your boob to read our book?
>
> The BOOB it's minus the bump in front
> because the doctor made it blunt with Mickey.
> She'll forever lean over to one side,
> She'll sway around just like the tide, don't tease her.
>
> She's our goofy, bubbly Tammy
> and she's fine.
> Came through those stupid awful treatments
> Come on all and have a good time.

Okay, so Dolly Parton doesn't have to worry about any songwriting competition, but it was the loving thought that really counted!!!

The "rag" I chose was one of my grandmothers hand-stitched quilt tops to share with everyone. I talked about all the things and people I was grateful for and it was a really sweet evening!

Lesson Twenty – Live life to the fullest! This book is about surviving cancer, but we are all survivors at one time in our lives. This may be an illness, or a bad relationship, the death of someone close, or a divorce, or any other life-changing situation. If we don't take the opportunity to live today, when will we find the time to do it later? There are no guarantees for any of us and we have to live each day to the fullest. Sometimes it means stepping outside your comfort zone, but you will find that with each step, your comfort zone gets larger and larger, and as the path gets wider and longer, life gets more exciting.

Chapter Twenty
Winning the Mind Game
The final chapter of this book – a mere preface to the rest of my life!

"God never promised us a calm passage, just a safe landing." — Unknown Author

Throughout this entire journey, I have learned many wonderful lessons; lessons that I have tried to share through the pages of this book. Now, the major thrust of this ordeal is seemingly over, but what is left is something that I think many people deal with on a daily basis – the mind game.

What I refer to as the "mind game" is the feeling that from this point forth in my life I will come back to the original diagnosis and think the smallest bump that I can't explain or the slightest scratch that doesn't seem to heal correctly will turn out to be cancer once again. That is one terrible condition of this dreaded disease – it seems as though we can try to keep it at bay, but some how it finds us. The scars from all the surgeries have healed nicely, and although they are a constant reminder of this journey, I have been blessed with a tremendous amount of wonderful events along the path, from the people I have met, and the experiences of each day. There is no explanation for most cancers, so what are we to do about this constant nagging in the back of our minds? I have a few suggestions (I know, you thought I would!).

First, let's review some of the information we examined in previous chapters. We have discussed the fact that our minds are wonderful things, but in reality our minds can only house one thought at a time. Here we are, back at making choices in life. I find this very difficult to get started at times, but then I stop and remind myself of this fact.

I get an ache or pain, a bump or bruise and, when my mind quickly goes to what it "could be", I try very hard to re-focus and turn the thoughts back to my "I am healthy" mantra, or simply repeating positive words. I also find this to be a greater challenge if I am sitting and doing nothing. Okay, okay, for those of you who know me, you know this RARELY happens, but every now and then... In those times, I have to try even harder to bring my thoughts back to the positive and get rid of the negative thoughts. And, I know I have to get busy doing SOMETHING – anything to keep me out of the dark and despair. I suggest that you occupy your mind with something great and you will see a huge difference on your horizon.

Just recently I was listening to a set of motivational tapes, and the speaker was affirming the idea that the brain can only house one thought at a time, and we have a choice. He also said that the strange thing about the subconscious is that it will work on any information that we give it – positive or negative. Think about that for a minute. If we can control what our mind thinks, as we have discussed many times in this book, how much easier is it for us to think of a pleasant thought – a bright sunny day with lots of colors and flowers, for example, or the cool feel of the sand beneath our bare feet as we walk along the ocean shore.

I have talked with other people about this mind game, and it certainly isn't a game that only cancer survivors tend to play. Of the people I have talked with who have suffered other ailments, disappointments, or tragic experiences, the response seems to be the same. The mind tries to take you to places you do not want to go and you have to lasso it, pull it back, and focus on the positive.

The funny image I have in my head right now is from the movie "9 to 5" with Dolly Parton (of course, I would bring her back in – you know she's one of my favorites), Lily Tomlin, and Jane Fonda. If you want to laugh, this is one movie I would recommend, especially if you work outside of the home in an office with others! It has some crazy parts, but some of the images are priceless as I replace the characters on the screen with some people in my own life! What a riot!

Anyway, back to the story line. In this movie there is a scene where Dolly is going around with her lasso and lassoing her boss who is a royal pain. The thought of the lasso brings me to the thinking that we can lasso this ugly monster of negative thought, and squeeze it down – in fact, squeeze it down until it disappears into nothing! Then re-paint the scenery in the way we choose.

In April 2003, I was honored to be asked to speak at a "Survivors Conference" for the American Cancer Society. Shortly before the conference, in fact at 11 PM the night before the conference, I received a phone call from Dr. B telling me that my recent mammogram showed suspicious shadows and we might be going back into surgery again. Although I certainly wasn't "excited" about this prospect, this second time around my whole attitude and demeanor were apparently different; at least that is what I was told by some of my closest friends. I think it was the idea that I knew better what to expect this time. I wasn't afraid of facing radiation as I was before. I knew much better what to expect as far as healing time was concerned. I had a better idea of what to expect from long range healing regarding scars, but most importantly, I already had my mantra in place and I knew that I was and AM a survivor! As it turned out, we did a surgical biopsy but there was no cancer (thank God!). The fear of the unknown can be so powerful, but the positive thoughts and the idea that I knew what to expect, pulled me through not only this second ordeal, but the many times after this episode that I felt that mysterious bump or bruise.

There was a commercial on television sometime ago that ended with, "The mind is a terrible thing to waste". I would agree whole heartedly. In fact, I would add that the thoughts we put in our minds are very powerful – we don't even realize the extreme power of our thoughts, or what we can do with them to change our lives in enormous ways. There are so many examples out there of people visualizing great success and achieving exactly what they visualized. I think that is sometimes the most difficult, but essential part – being able to REALLY see ourselves healthy again.

I know that having gone through this I view the world in a totally different way than I did before September 2001 – in most ways it is a much better idea of the world around me. I have learned so very much while walking this journey. I have learned that there are people who care deeply for me. I have learned that each day is a gift. I have learned that there are many things in this world that cannot be explained, from one end of the spectrum to the other - I don't know why I got cancer (the seemingly negative end of the spectrum) and I had no idea the joy or thankfulness I could feel as I sensed the many miracles (call them what you will – I like miracles) that have surrounded my life since that time (the most positive end of the spectrum).

Make the choice – make it your choice – you have one thought at a time in that pretty little head of yours – make it the right thought – the encouraging, upbeat, motivating, encouraging (whatever words you choose to use) thought – your choice!!!

There have been so many blessings on this journey that I would NEVER have expected when I was first told by Dr. G that he was suspecting cancer. I have met fantastic people and had incredible experiences. It reminds me of a saying that I have hanging on my office wall that I see daily. I do not know the author, but perhaps it will help you at some point, too:

The man whispered, "God, speak to me"
And a meadowlark sang.
But, the man did not hear.

So the man yelled "God, speak to me!"
And, the thunder rolled across the sky.
But, the man did not listen.

The man looked around and said,
"God let me see you"
And a star shined brightly.
But, the man did not notice.

And, the man shouted,
"God show me a miracle!"
And, a life was born.
But, the man did not know.

So, the man cried out in despair,
"Touch me God, and let me know you are here!"
Whereupon, God reached down and touched the man.
But, the man brushed the
butterfly away and walked on.

Don't miss out on a blessing because it isn't
packaged the way that you expect.

Final Thoughts

In closing this book, may I leave you with some final thoughts. Life and the people in it are blessings to enjoy, cherish, and embrace. May you find your path to recovery filled with many of these blessings, and may you daily take time to laugh, as it is the music of the soul.

As you always look for the Lighter Side of Recovery (and LIFE), may God bless your path to healing, in ways you never thought possible.

Many blessing to you on your journey!

Whew!! Now that the book is done - it is time for another party!!! Now, where did I put those clown noses and feather boa again.......

> Dear Lord, please use me this day
> beyond my wildest dreams!

Appendix
Suggested Questions

Throughout this journey there were so many questions to ask. As I indicated before, there are a lot of personal decisions that one has to make on this journey. My theory is that if you don't know the answers to your questions, you will be unable to make some of these important decisions. For many, the questions they should be asking are the hard part. There is so much happening so quickly that you aren't even sure where to begin.

This section is designed to help start your question asking, and spark you on to asking other questions as needed. The list includes my own personal questions and a few I picked up along the way. Whatever questions you choose – just don't be afraid to ASK!!!

I apologized to Dr. B once for asking so many questions (I wasn't REALLY sorry, but it seemed like the right thing to say). He immediately told me that he "prefers" it when patients come in with their questions. He said if his patients don't ask questions, he has no way of knowing what they need to know. Makes sense to me.

Since I have traveled this path, two very close friends have faced similar situations. I truly believe that everything in our lives happens for a reason. In these particular cases, I was able to help these friends by offering some good basic information, an understanding ear, and some direction on what can be a very scary path.

When you are diagnosed with something that can ultimately be life threatening, your whole life seemingly slows down and you feel like you are observing everything happening from some sort of haze. Hopefully, these suggested questions will be helpful on your quest for answers.

It is my recommendation that you mark these pages and take the book with you to your first office visit after being diagnosed. As I mentioned before, using a video camera can be very helpful when you return home and have all of the questions and answers floating around in your head. I truly do not believe that most doctors intend on talking "over the patient's head", but make sure you are asking for very specific definitions to terms you do not understand. If you are unfortunate enough to get a doctor who is impatient with your questions, don't just settle for that type of response – hold that person accountable and GET THE ANSWERS - this is <u>your</u> life.

Mammogram shows a possible problem

1. What <u>specifically</u> makes you think there is a problem?

2. What do we do now?

3. If a needle biopsy is an option, and it comes back negative (no cancer indicated), how certain are we that it is accurate?

4. If the biopsy comes back positive (cancer indicated), what are my options? On what are you basing these options (ask for specific studies, etc.)?

5. Who reads the mammogram? Is it by a person and machine to double check accuracy?

Further tests confirm there is some type of cancer

1. What do we do now? What tests? What are we looking for? How accurate are these follow-up tests?

2. What do we do next?

3. What is the name of the cancer that I have? (There are different types of breast cancer so make sure you know exactly what type you are facing. The different types dictate the path of treatment.)

4. Ask you doctor for a book with good information about breast cancer. The National Institute of Health publishes an excellent, very informative book that can be used as a reference. Take it with you and have the doctor mark exactly what he/she is recommending.

5. How large was the tumor?

6. Do you expect to find any cancer in the lymph nodes?

7. What other tests do we do right now to make sure the cancer is not located any place in my body?

8. What is the difference between a lumpectomy and mastectomy?

9. What determines whether we do a lumpectomy or mastectomy, and from what you see, what are you thinking at this time? What are the advantages and disadvantages of each surgery?

10. What can I expect my breast to look like after this type of surgery?

11. What about reconstruction? Can it be done at the same time as the lumpectomy or mastectomy?

12. How long will I be in the hospital?

13. How long will I be off work? Will there be any restrictions?

14. What type of follow-up do you recommend (radiation, chemotherapy, and other options)?

15. Since there has been time lapse since the initial mammogram, how much time do I have to make a decision?

16. Are there people you can recommend that I can talk with who have been through similar situations?

17. Do you recommend any books or materials for me to read?

18. Where can I contact support groups in this area?

19. If I have additional questions, how can I contact you or your nurse?

20. How do I get a full copy of my records?

Thoughts for after the surgery and into recovery

1. If Tamoxifen is recommended – what are the benefits and how do you think this compares to the newer medications like Anastrozole (Arimidex), or others that may be available?

2. Higher risk for osteoporosis and heart disease and cholesterol– are there baseline tests we do so we have something to compare to in the future? What are your views on Evista at this point?

3. What exercises can I do to strengthen the arm without risking lymphedema?

4. What are your thoughts on hot flashes – Clonidine – high blood pressure vs. Effexor?

5. What is the long-term follow-up schedule? (Every 3 months, 6 months, etc.)

6. What types of things should I report to you in the meantime?

7. Are there any dietary concerns?

Oncology Questions

1. What type of treatments will I receive (chemotherapy, hormonal, or immunotherapy)? What is the difference and why this treatment?

2. How do you know what best drugs for ME?

3. I understand you may do tests to check my heart and other organs before starting treatments. What are they, why, and when will they be done?

4. Do you use or recommend Zofran for the nausea? Standard or on my request?

5. Can I take Tylenol for head or backache while on chemo?

6. How long will this last – how many injections? What are my choices? Should I have an I.V. port?

7. Am I a candidate for ovarian ablation? What are your views on this procedure?

8. I understand one risk of the treatments I will be receiving is early menopause – what exactly does that mean?

9. How long does chemo stay in your system? How does it come out?

10. When do I start Tamoxifen? With Tamoxifen will I be able to take estrogen to lessen hot flashes, etc. (if I wanted to) for the menopausal side effects?

11. How will we know the drugs are working? I usually don't need full prescription dosages – does that have a bearing on this treatment?

12. What side effects should I report immediately to you and how can I reach you after hours in an emergency?

13. Are there any restrictions at all? (Example – exercise (most brisk walking), flossing, etc.)?

14. Anything I can do in preparation of the treatments? (I have already had a flu shot and all dental work done.)

15. Can I get a massage? Are you familiar with massage used in conjunction with chemo to lesson the side effects?

16. If you currently take vitamins, is there any reason to stop them during this treatment?

Radiology Questions

1. How will the dosage (both length of time and strength) be determined and by whom?

2. What will I wear when I am radiated?

3. What type of privacy does this facility offer to the patients?

4. Will this be internal or external and why? What are the options and differences?

5. What is actually being radiated (breast and lymph nodes)? Do you anticipate any problems with either?

6. Will there be any permanent effects of this treatment (for example, permanent numbness in the arm, higher risk of cancer in the radiated area due to the treatment, or higher risk or pneumonia)?

7. What is the role of my surgeon and oncologist in this treatment?

8. What steps do you take to protect my other organs, especially the heart?

9. How often do I see the actual doctor when I have the radiation treatments?

10. What types of things should I report immediately to the doctor or therapist? What side effects should I expect? What can I do to avoid or eliminate them?

11. Will I have any tests in conjunction with the radiation treatments (EKG, blood drawn, etc.)? If so, what are they are why are they being requested?

12. How do you gauge any progress or change? How do you know it is working?

13. Do you recommend any extra types of vitamins during the treatment?

14. When will I have the "simulation" (the initial markings on the body for the radiation treatments)? How long will the process take?

15. Are the permanent tattoos absolutely necessary? If recommended, how large will they be and where?

16. How will my breast look after the treatments?

17. Are there any restrictions to my daily activities?

18. What type of follow-up schedule should I expect?

References

This section lists in alphabetical order some web sites and books that I found helpful on my journey. Some were helpful in answering questions that I had and others helped me develop questions to ask my doctors. Other books on the list offered encouragement and guidance on the journey. You may find this list helpful, or not, but I would like to suggest that you look at these and other references to help yourself make informed decisions on your personal path to recovery.

Web Sites:

http://www.breastcancer.org (A non-profit organization for breast cancer education)

http://www.cancer.org (Home page for the American Cancer Society)

www.elsevier.com/locate/radonline (Radiation and Oncology Journal on line for technical journal articles)

http://health.nih.gov (National Institutes of Health site – a great deal of information on a lot of different diseases and treatments. There are also a number of very informative booklets that you can order or download in their entirety from this site through the CancerNet at: http://cancer.gov/cancerinformation)

www.hystersisters.com (A site devoted to issues associated with hysterectomies)

http://www.komen.org (The Susan G. Komen Breast Cancer Foundation page – a lot of good, basic information about cancer research and ways you can get involved) http://www.natlbcc.org (National Breast Cancer Coalition – a national advocacy and education group)

http://www.nccn.org (National Comprehensive Cancer Network - an alliance of 19 of the world's leading cancer centers, is an authoritative source of information to help patients and health professionals make informed decisions about cancer care.)

www.toastmasters.org (An International organization devoted to helping people develop effective communication skills)

Books:

Norman Cousins. *Anatomy of an Illness as Perceived by the Patient: Reflections on Healing and Regeneration*, W. W. Norton & Company, 1979.

Judy C. Kneece. *Your Breast Cancer Treatment Book.* EduCare Publishing, P. O. Box 280305, Columbia, SC 29228, 1-803-796-6100, 1995

Norman Vincent Peale, *In God We Trust: A Positive Faith for Troubled Times.* Thomas Nelson Publishers, 1994.

Zig Ziglar. *Staying Up, Up Up in a Down, Down World: Daily Hope for the Daily Grind.* Thomas Nelson Publishers, 2000.

Breast Cancer: Treatment Guidelines for Patients. This is the booklet in which Dr. B "highlighted" all of the information pertaining to my diagnosis and treatment options. I found it very helpful and straight forward. This booklet is presented through a partnership with the American Cancer Society and the National Comprehensive Cancer Network.

There are a number of booklets available through the National Cancer Institute (NCI). Topics include a wide range of subject matter including basic cancer information, treatments options, and recovery information. You can start by calling 1-800-4-CANCER, or by going to the NCI website at:

http://cancer.gov/cancerinfo/ and go to the "Cancer Literature" information section.

Red Nose Fund

I hope that you have found this book to be helpful as you or someone you love travel down the path to recovery. If you would like to make a donation to a fund designated to offset printing costs, so that copies of this book may be donated to patients and breast care centers, please contact:

Tammy A. Miller
530 Hillside Ave
State College, PA 16803
(814) 360-4031 or
(814) 231-3001
E-Mail: **tammy@hugzandcompany.com**

Bulk sales discounts are available. Please contact the author at the above information for further details.

Need A Speaker?

Are you looking for a speaker or workshop for your next event? Contact Tammy at:

>Hugz and Company Consulting
>*"Leaders in Learning and Laughter"*
>
>530 Hillside Ave.
>State College, PA 16803
>
>(814) 360-4031 or
>(814) 231-3001
>
>E-mail: tammy@hugzandcompany.com

The following are examples of some of the workshops presented by Hugz & Company Consulting

>**The Lighter Side of Recovery: Lessons Learned Along the Path**
>
>**Brain Aerobics**
>
>**The Magic of Motivation**
>
>**Embracing a Successful Attitude**
>
>**This Funny Place Called Work**
>
>**Winning Presentation Styles**
>
>**Discovering the Clown Within**

The Lighter Side of Recovery: Lessons Learned Along the Path

The value of humor in healing is still a relatively new topic of research. In this lively presentation, we examine how we can use humor to help us heal in even the most serious of health issues. As a cancer survivor, Tammy discusses the "Lessons Learned Along the Path", but her path to recovery may not be the path you expect. This lighthearted approach to healing is a healthy reminder to all of us that life is about choices, and we have many more choices that we realize.

Brain Aerobics

The human brain is a mysterious and largely undiscovered organ that makes us who we are. Until recently, it was thought that the brain lost its capability as we aged. Recent discoveries have shown that the brain can be exercised, strengthened, and grown no matter how old we are. In this session, you will learn how to unleash your creative self, tailor an exercise regimen for your brain, and enhance your learning skills through game playing, mind-mapping, and bringing out the kid in you!

The Magic of Motivation

Stuck in a rut and looking for a ladder to help you climb out? Want to discover why some people seem to have it all together and others are still trying to find the pieces? In this enlightening and entertaining workshop, you will discover the tools necessary to create your own personal ladder to success. By examining the roles of motivation, self-esteem, and positive attitude, you will learn how to add passion, pleasure, and purpose to every aspect of your life.

Embracing a Successful Attitude

Choosing the right attitude can make a major difference in our lives both at work and at home. This workshop helps you to recognize the attitude choices you currently make, and how you can change the directional path you have chosen, for greater success. This lighthearted presentation offers practical steps to making changes, developing your strengths, and identifying your weaknesses. Join the fun and learn along the way.

This Funny Place Called Work

This workshop will look at the benefits of taking your job seriously, but yourself lightly. This upbeat session looks at ways to bring humor to your work place on a daily basis. Through lively discussions and hands on activities, you will find a variety of ways to enjoy the day while getting the work done. You will learn how to look for humor, sometimes creating your own, but always finding an excuse to laugh.

Guide to Winning Presentations

Making an effective presentation involves much more than just getting in front of an audience and speaking. This workshop will teach you the very basics you need to deliver a winning presentation. Learn how to structure your presentation, adapt your message to a specific audience, bring vocal variety and body language to your delivery, help ease your stage fright, and make use of other presentation skills that will make your audience sit up and listen.

Discovering the Clown Within

Everyone loves the circus and the clowns who make them laugh. In this session, you will learn the basics of clowning, including the history, types, and styles of clowns. You'll be shown how to develop your own personal character, apply make-up, design a costume, create balloon animals, make props from household items, and perform simple magic. Whether you want to run away and join the circus, just entertain children, or anything in between, this will get you started in this fascinating world of fun and excitement.

Also available from Lighthearted Press:

*The Joyful Journey of Hospital Clowning:
Making a Difference With Love and Laughter*
New 2003 Edition

"This is a great book." — Dr. Richard Snowberg

Photo Section

by Tiffany Earnest, Tiffany Dawn Designs
www.tiffanydawndesigns.com

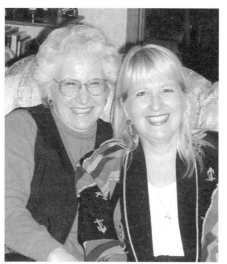
Tammy and Mom

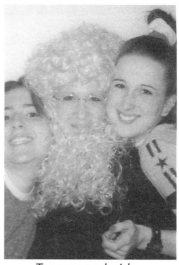
Tammy and girls

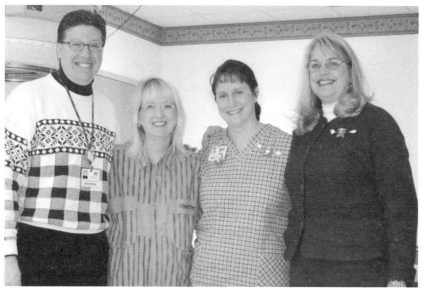
The radiology morning team

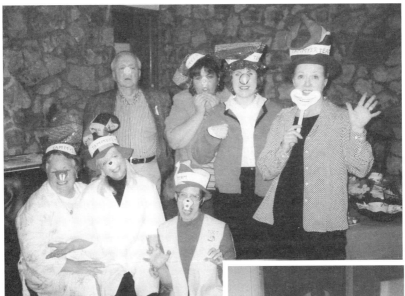

Humor team at the "Wild Party"

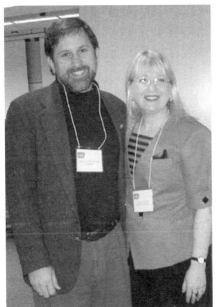

Tammy and Dr. B

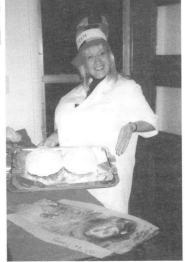

The Wild Party Keeping Abreast!

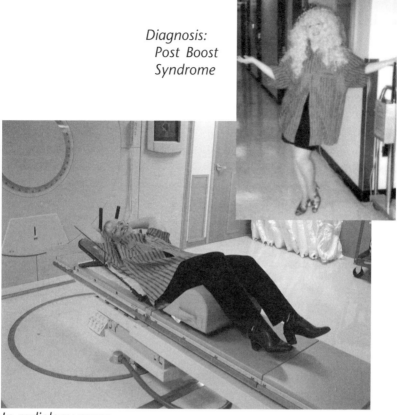

Diagnosis: Post Boost Syndrome

In radiology room

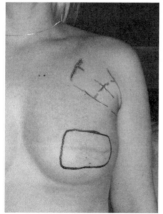

Radiation markings

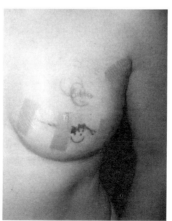

Artwork by Dr. B

Notes

Notes